Underground Clinical Vignettes

Neurology

FOURTH EDITION

Underground
Clinical Vignettes
Neurology

FOURTH EDITION

Sandra I. Kim, M.D., Ph.D.
Resident in Internal Medicine
Beth Israel Deaconess Medical Center
Harvard Medical School
Boston, Massachusetts

Todd A. Swanson, M.D., Ph.D.
Resident in Radiation Oncology
William Beaumont Hospital
Royal Oak, Michigan

Nadeem N. Hussain, M.D.
Fellow in Psychiatry
University of Illinois Medical Center
Chicago, Illinois

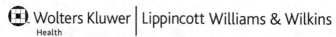
Wolters Kluwer | Lippincott Williams & Wilkins
Health
Philadelphia · Baltimore · New York · London
Buenos Aires · Hong Kong · Sydney · Tokyo

MT

Acquisitions editor: Nancy Anastasi Duffy
Developmental editor: Nancy Hoffmann
Managing editor: Kelly Horvath
Associate Production manager: Kevin P. Johnson
Marketing manager: Jennifer Kuklinski
Creative Director: Doug Smock
Compositor: International Typesetting and Composition

© 2007 by Lippincott Williams & Wilkins
UCV Step 2 *Neurology*, Fourth Edition

Lippincott Williams & Wilkins, a Wolters Kluwer business.

351 West Camden Street   530 Walnut Street
Baltimore, MD 21201   Philadelphia, PA 19106

9 8 7 6 5 4 3 2 1

Library of Congress Cataloging-in-Publication Data
Kim, Sandra.
    Neurology.—4th ed. / Sandra I. Kim, Todd A. Swanson, Nadeem N. Hussain.
        p. ; cm.—(Underground clinical vignettes)
    Rev. ed. of: Neurology / Vikhas Bhushan . . . [et al.]. 3rd ed. c2005.
    Includes index.
    ISBN 0-7817-6837-3
    1. Neurology—Case studies.   2. Physicians—Licenses—United States—Examinations—Study guides.
I. Swanson, Todd A.   II. Hussain, Nadeem N.   III. Neurology.   IV. Title.   V. Series.
    [DNLM: 1. Nervous System Diseases—Case Reports.   2. Nervous System Diseases—Problems
and Exercises.   WL 18.2 K497n 2007]
    RC359.B57 2007
    616.80076—dc22

                                                                    2007033865

DISCLAIMER

5/9/11

dedication

Dedicated to Sajjad Hussain, Omar Hussain, and Sameena Wafa.

preface

First published in 1999, the Underground Clinical Vignettes series has provided thousands of students with a highly effective review tool as they prepare for medical exams, particularly the USMLE Step 1 and 2 exams. Designed as a quick study guide, each UCV book contains patient-centered clinical cases that highlight a range of medical diagnoses.

With this new edition of *Step 2 Underground Clinical Vignettes,* we have incorporated feedback from medical students across the country to provide updated cases with expanded treatment and discussion sections. Every title has more cases, drawing from a broader area within each discipline. A new two-page format enables readers to formulate an initial diagnosis before reading the answer to each case. The inclusion of relevant MRI images, X-rays, and photographs allows students to more readily visualize the physical presentation of each case. Breakout boxes, tables, and algorithms have been added, along with 20 all-new, Board-format QAs, making this edition of UCV an ideal source of information for exam review, classroom discussion, and clinical rotations.

The clinical vignettes in this Step 2 series have been revised and updated to reflect current medical thinking on medication, pathogenesis, epidemiology, management, and complications. Although each case presents most of the signs, symptoms, and diagnostic findings for a particular illness, patients typically will not present with such a "complete" picture either clinically or on a medical examination. Cases are not meant to simulate a potential real patient or an exam vignette.

Access to LWW's online companion site, ThePoint, will be offered as a premium with the purchase of the Underground Clinical Vignettes Step 2 bundle. Benefits include an online test link and 160 additional new Board-format questions covering all UCV subject areas.

We hope you will find the Underground Clinical Vignettes series informative and useful. We welcome any feedback, suggestions, or corrections you have about this series. Please contact us at LWW.com/medstudent.

preface

contributors

Series Editors

Sandra I. Kim, M.D., Ph.D.
Resident in Internal Medicine
Beth Israel Deaconess Medical Center
Harvard Medical School
Boston, Massachusetts

Todd A. Swanson, M.D., Ph.D.
Resident in Radiation Oncology
William Beaumont Hospital
Royal Oak, Michigan

Book Editor

Nadeem N. Hussain, M.D.
Fellow in Psychiatry
University of Illinois Medical Center
Chicago, Illinois

Contributing Editor

Trudy D. Pang, M.D.
Epilepsy Fellow in Neurology
Beth Israel Deaconess Medical Center
Harvard Medical School
Boston, Massachusetts

Neurology Contributors

Andrew Tarulli, M.D.
Meghan Delaney, M.D.
Andrew Z. Wang, M.D.
Asim Roy, M.D.
Swaminathan Karthik, M.D.
Amy N. H. Amick, M.D.

acknowledgments

Our great thanks to the house staff and faculty from Beth Israel Deaconess, Massachusetts General, Brigham and Women's, and Children's Hospitals in Boston, whose clinical cases, revisions, and suggestions were indispensable to this series. Thanks to the editors at Lippincott, especially Nancy Hoffmann, who worked overtime on these books.

abbreviations

A-a	alveolar-arterial (oxygen gradient)	ATLS	Advanced Trauma Life Support (protocol)
AAA	abdominal aortic aneurysm		
ABCs	airway, breathing, circulation	ATN	acute tubular necrosis
ABGs	arterial blood gases	ATPase	adenosine triphosphatase
ABPA	allergic bronchopulmonary aspergillosis	ATRA	all-*trans*-retinoic acid
		AV	arteriovenous, atrioventricular
ABVD	Adriamycin, bleomycin, vinblastine, dacarbazine (chemotherapy)	AVPD	avoidant personality disorder
		AXR	abdominal X-ray
ACE	angiotensin-converting enzyme	AZT	azidothymidine (zidovudine)
ACTH	adrenocorticotropic hormone	BCG	bacille Calmette-Guérin
ADA	adenosine deaminase, American Diabetic Association	BE	barium enema
		BP	blood pressure
ADH	antidiuretic hormone	BPD	borderline personality disorder
ADHD	attention-deficit hyperactivity disorder	BPH	benign prostatic hypertrophy
		BPK	B-cell progenitor kinase
AED	automatic external defibrillator	BPM	beats per minute
AFP	α-fetoprotein	BUN	blood urea nitrogen
AI	aortic insufficiency	CAA	cerebral amyloid angiopathy
AICD	automatic internal cardiac defibrillator	CABG	coronary artery bypass grafting
		CAD	coronary artery disease
AIDS	acquired immunodeficiency syndrome	CALLA	common acute lymphoblastic leukemia antigen
ALL	acute lymphocytic leukemia	C-ANCA	cytoplasmic antineutrophil cytoplasmic antibody
ALS	amyotrophic lateral sclerosis		
ALT	alanine aminotransferase	CAO	chronic airway obstruction
AML	acute myelogenous leukemia	CAP	community-acquired pneumonia
AMP	adenosine monophosphate	CBC	complete blood count
ANA	antinuclear antibody	CBD	common bile duct
ANCA	antineutrophil cytoplasmic antibody	CBT	cognitive behavioral therapy
		CCU	cardiac care unit
Angio	angiography	CD	cluster of differentiation
AP	anteroposterior	CDC	Centers for Disease Control
aPTT	activated partial thromboplastin time	CEA	carcinoembryonic antigen
		CF	cystic fibrosis
ARDS	adult respiratory distress syndrome	CFTR	cystic fibrosis transmembrane regulator
ARF	acute renal failure	CFU	colony-forming unit
AS	ankylosing spondylitis	CHF	congestive heart failure
ASA	acetylsalicylic acid	CJD	Creutzfeldt–Jakob disease
5-ASA	5-aminosalicylic acid	CK	creatine kinase
ASD	atrial septal defect	CK-MB	creatine kinase, MB fraction
ASO	antistreptolysin O	CLL	chronic lymphocytic leukemia
AST	aspartate aminotransferase	CML	chronic myelogenous leukemia

CMV	cytomegalovirus	EMG	electromyography
CN	cranial nerve	ER	emergency room
CNS	central nervous system	ERCP	endoscopic retrograde cholan-
CO	cardiac output		giopancreatography
COPD	chronic obstructive pulmonary	ESR	erythrocyte sedimentation rate
	disease	EtOH	ethanol
CPAP	continuous positive airway	FDA	Food and Drug Administration
	pressure	Fe_{Na}	fractional excretion of sodium
CPK	creatine phosphokinase	FEV1	forced expiratory volume in 1
CPR	cardiopulmonary resuscitation		second
CRP	C-reactive protein	FIGO	International Federation of
CSF	cerebrospinal fluid		Gynecology and Obstetrics
CT	computed tomography		(classification)
CVA	cerebrovascular accident	FIO_2	fraction of inspired oxygen
CXR	chest X-ray	FNA	fine-needle aspiration
D&C	dilatation and curettage	FRC	functional residual capacity
DAF	decay-accelerating factor	FSH	follicle-stimulating hormone
DC	direct current	FTA	fluorescent treponemal antibody
DEXA	dual-energy X-ray absorptiometry	FTA-ABS	fluorescent treponemal antibody
DHEA	dehydroepiandrosterone		absorption test
DIC	disseminated intravascular	5-FU	5-fluorouracil
	coagulation	FVC	forced vital capacity
DIP	distal interphalangeal (joint)	G6PD	glucose-6-phosphate dehydroge-
DKA	diabetic ketoacidosis		nase
DLCO	diffusing capacity of carbon	GA	gestational age
	monoxide	GABA	gamma-aminobutyric acid
DM	diabetes mellitus	GABHS	group A β-hemolytic streptococcus
DMD	Duchenne's muscular dystrophy	GAD	generalized anxiety disorder
DNA	deoxyribonucleic acid	GBM	glomerular basement membrane
DNase	deoxyribonuclease	G-CSF	granulocyte colony-stimulating
dsDNA	double-stranded DNA		factor
DTP	diphtheria, tetanus, pertussis	GERD	gastroesophageal reflux disease
	(vaccine)	GFR	glomerular filtration rate
DTRs	deep tendon reflexes	GGT	gamma-glutamyltransferase
DTs	delirium tremens	GI	gastrointestinal
DUB	dysfunctional uterine bleeding	GnRH	gonadotropin-releasing hormone
DVT	deep venous thrombosis	GU	genitourinary
EBV	Epstein–Barr virus	HAV	hepatitis A virus
ECG	electrocardiography	Hb	hemoglobin
Echo	echocardiography	HBcAg	hepatitis B core antigen
ECMO	extracorporeal membrane	HBsAg	hepatitis B surface antigen
	oxygenation	HBV	hepatitis B virus
EDTA	ethylenediamine tetraacetic acid	hCG	human chorionic gonadotropin
EEG	electroencephalography	HCl	hydrogen chloride
EF	ejection fraction	HCO_3	bicarbonate
EGD	esophagogastroduodenoscopy	Hct	hematocrit
E:I	expiratory-to-inspiratory (ratio)	HCV	hepatitis C virus
ELISA	enzyme-linked immunosorbent	HDL	high-density lipoprotein
	assay	HEENT	head, eyes, ears, nose, and
EM	electron microscopy		throat

HELLP	hemolysis, elevated liver enzymes, low platelets (syndrome)	KUB	kidney, ureter, bladder
HEV	hepatitis E virus	LA	left atrium
HGPRT	hypoxanthine-guanine phospho-ribosyltransferase	LAMB	lentigines, atrial myxoma, blue nevi (syndrome)
HHV	human herpesvirus	LD	Leishman-Donovan (body)
5-HIAA	5-hydroxyindoleacetic acid	LDH	lactate dehydrogenase
HIDA	hepato-iminodiacetic acid (scan)	LDL	low-density lipoprotein
HIV	human immunodeficiency virus	LES	lower esophageal sphincter
HLA	human leukocyte antigen	LFTs	liver function tests
HPF	high-power field	LH	luteinizing hormone
HPI	history of present illness	LHRH	luteinizing hormone–releasing hormone
HPV	human papillomavirus	LKM	liver-kidney microsomal (antibody)
HR	heart rate	LMN	lower motor neuron
HRCT	high-resolution computed tomography	LP	lumbar puncture
HS	hereditary spherocytosis	L/S	lecithin-to-sphingomyelin (ratio)
HSG	hysterosalpingography	LSD	lysergic acid diethylamide
HSV	herpes simplex virus	LV	left ventricle, left ventricular
HUS	hemolytic-uremic syndrome	LVH	left ventricular hypertrophy
IABC	intra-aortic balloon counterpul-sation	Lytes	electrolytes
ICA	internal carotid artery	Mammo	mammography
ICD	implantable cardiac defibrillator	MAO	monoamine oxidase (inhibitor)
ICP	intracranial pressure	MAP	mean arterial pressure
ICU	intensive care unit	MCA	middle cerebral artery
ID/CC	identification and chief complaint	MCHC	mean corpuscular hemoglobin concentration
IDDM	insulin-dependent diabetes mellitus	MCP	metacarpophalangeal (joint)
IE	infectious endocarditis	MCV	mean corpuscular volume
IFA	immunofluorescent antibody	MDMA	3,4-methylene-dioxymetham-phetamine ("Ecstasy")
Ig	immunoglobulin	MEN	multiple endocrine neoplasia
IL	interleukin	MGUS	monoclonal gammopathy of undetermined origin
IM	infectious mononucleosis, intramuscular	MHC	major histocompatibility complex
INH	isoniazid	MI	myocardial infarction
INR	International Normalized Ratio	MIBG	metaiodobenzylguanidine
123-ISS	iodine-123-labeled somatostatin	MMR	measles, mumps, rubella (vaccine)
IUD	intrauterine device	MPTP	1-methyl-4-phenyl-tetrahydropy-ridine
IUGR	intrauterine growth retardation	MR	magnetic resonance (imaging)
IV	intravenous	mRNA	messenger ribonucleic acid
IVC	inferior vena cava	MRSA	methicillin-resistant *Staphylococcus aureus*
IVIG	intravenous immunoglobulin	MS	multiple sclerosis
IVP	intravenous pyelography	MTP	metatarsophalangeal (joint)
JRA	juvenile rheumatoid arthritis	MuSK	muscle-specific kinase
JVD	jugular venous distention	MVA	motor vehicle accident
JVP	jugular venous pressure	NADPH	reduced nicotinamide adenine dinucleotide phosphate
KOH	potassium hydroxide		
KS	Kaposi's sarcoma		

NAME	nevi, atrial myxoma, myxoid neurofibroma, ephilides (syndrome)
NG	nasogastric
NIDDM	noninsulin-dependent diabetes mellitus
NMDA	N-methyl-D-aspartate
NPO	nil per os (nothing by mouth)
NSAID	nonsteroidal anti-inflammatory drug
Nuc	nuclear medicine
OCD	obsessive-compulsive disorder
OCP	oral contraceptive pill
OCPD	obsessive-compulsive personality disorder
17-OHP	17-hydroxyprogesterone
OPC	organophosphate and carbamate
OS	opening snap
OTC	over the counter
PA	posteroanterior
2-PAM	pralidoxime
P-ANCA	perinuclear antineutrophil cytoplasmic antibody
Pao_2	partial pressure of oxygen
PAS	periodic acid Schiff
PBS	peripheral blood smear
PCO_2	partial pressure of carbon dioxide
PCOD	polycystic ovary disease
PCP	phencyclidine
PCR	polymerase chain reaction
PCV	polycythemia vera
PDA	patent ductus arteriosus
PE	physical exam
PEEP	positive end-expiratory pressure
PET	positron emission tomography
PFTs	pulmonary function tests
PID	pelvic inflammatory disease
PIP	proximal interphalangeal (joint)
PKU	phenylketonuria
PMI	point of maximal impulse
PMN	polymorphonuclear (leukocyte)
PO	per os (by mouth)
Po_2	partial pressure of oxygen
PPD	purified protein derivative
PROM	premature rupture of membranes
PRPP	phosphoribosyl pyrophosphate
PSA	prostate-specific antigen
PT	prothrombin time
PTE	pulmonary thromboembolism
PTH	parathyroid hormone
PTSD	posttraumatic stress disorder
PTT	partial thromboplastin time
RA	rheumatoid arthritis, right atrial
RBC	red blood cell
RDW	red-cell distribution width
REM	rapid eye movement
RF	rheumatoid factor
RhoGAM	Rh immune globulin
RNA	ribonucleic acid
RPR	rapid plasma reagin
RR	respiratory rate
RS	Reed-Sternberg (cell)
RSV	respiratory syncytial virus
RTA	renal tubular acidosis
RUQ	right upper quadrant
RV	residual volume, right ventricle, right ventricular
RVH	right ventricular hypertrophy
SA	sinoatrial
SAH	subarachnoid hemorrhage
Sao_2	oxygen saturation in arterial blood
SBE	subacute bacterial endocarditis
SBFT	small bowel follow-through
SC	subcutaneous
SCC	squamous cell carcinoma
SIADH	syndrome of inappropriate secretion of antidiuretic hormone
SIDS	sudden infant death syndrome
SLE	systemic lupus erythematosus
SMA	smooth muscle antibody
SSPE	subacute sclerosing panencephalitis
SSRI	selective serotonin reuptake inhibitor
STD	sexually transmitted disease
SZPD	schizoid personality disorder
T_3	triiodothyronine
T_4	thyroxine
TAB	therapeutic abortion
TB	tuberculosis
TBSA	total body surface area
TCA	tricyclic antidepressant
TCD	transcranial Doppler
TD	tardive dyskinesia
TENS	transcutaneous electrical nerve stimulation
TFTs	thyroid function tests
THC	*trans*-tetrahydrocannabinol
TIA	transient ischemic attack
TIBC	total iron-binding capacity

TIPS	transjugular intrahepatic portosystemic shunt	URI	upper respiratory infection
TLC	total lung capacity	US	ultrasound
TMJ	temporomandibular joint (syndrome)	UTI	urinary tract infection
		UV	ultraviolet
TMP-SMX	trimethoprim-sulfamethoxazole	VCUG	voiding cystourethrogram
TNF	tumor necrosis factor	VDRL	Venereal Disease Research Laboratory
TNM	tumor, node, metastasis (staging)		
ToRCH	*Toxoplasma,* rubella, CMV, herpes zoster	VF	ventricular fibrillation
		VIN	vulvar intraepithelial neoplasia
tPA	tissue plasminogen activator	VLDL	very low density lipoprotein
TPO	thyroid peroxidase	VMA	vanillylmandelic acid
TRAP	tartrate-resistant acid phosphatase	V/Q	ventilation-perfusion (ratio)
TRH	thyrotropin-releasing hormone	VS	vital signs
TSH	thyroid-stimulating hormone	VSD	ventricular septal defect
TSS	toxic shock syndrome	VT	ventricular tachycardia
TSST	toxic shock syndrome toxin	vWF	von Willebrand factor
TTP	thrombotic thrombocytopenic purpura	VZIG	varicella-zoster immune globulin
TUBD	transurethral balloon dilatation	VZV	varicella-zoster virus
TUIP	transurethral incision of the prostate	WAGR	Wilms' tumor, aniridia, ambiguous genitalia, mental retardation (syndrome)
TURP	transurethral resection of the prostate		
		WBC	white blood cell
UA	urinalysis	WG	Wegener's granulomatosis
UGI	upper GI (series)	WPW	Wolff–Parkinson–White (syndrome)
UMN	upper motor neuron		
		XR	X-ray

Underground Clinical Vignettes

Vignettes

Neurology

FOURTH EDITION

ID/CC　A **30-year-old woman** complains of gradual diminution of vision in the right eye.

HPI　She has had several **prior neurologic symptoms**, including an episode of loss of sensation and tingling in her left leg 1 year ago that lasted 2 to 3 days; she did not seek medical attention at that time. She has noted a gradual decrease of vision in her right eye over the last week, with discomfort on moving the right eye.

PE　VS: normal. PE: nystagmus; unable to adduct eyes on lateral gaze (internuclear ophthalmoplegia); swollen right optic nerve (due to optic neuritis) with blurred margins; visual acuity 20/400 in right eye and 20/20 in left eye; **DTRs asymmetrically hyperactive;** sensory and cerebellar exam intact; upon flexion of neck, she reports feeling "electric shocks" down her spine (LHERMITTE'S SIGN); symptoms worsen in a hot shower or bath (UHTHOFF'S SIGN).

Labs　LP: CSF shows **lymphocytic pleocytosis, oligoclonal bands** (most specific lab abnormality), elevated myelin basic protein, and negative Lyme titer. Impaired visual, auditory, and somatosensory evoked responses.

Imaging　MR, brain: **multiple periventricular white matter lesions** on T2-weighted image (see Fig. 1-1). MR, spine: large hyperintense plaque of demyelination at C5 level (see Fig. 1-2).

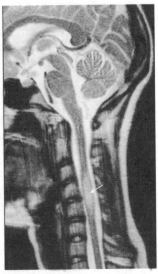

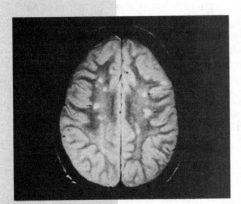

Figure 1-1. See imaging caption.

Figure 1-2. See imaging section.

case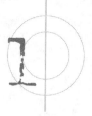

Multiple Sclerosis

Pathogenesis

Multiple sclerosis (MS) is probably an autoimmune process triggered by a virus (via molecular mimicry) occurring in a genetically susceptible person. The specific pathology is **demyelination** with axonal sparing. Any area of the CNS may be involved, but lesions commonly occur in the **lateral ventricular margins** of the **fourth ventricle.**

Epidemiology

Mean age of onset is 32 years, with a female-to-male ratio of 2 to 1; 25% of patients have a **family history.** Frequency rate **declines with increasing proximity to the equator.**

Management

Beta-interferon may be given to prevent recurrences in patients with relapsing MS. **Corticosteroids** are used for the treatment of acute relapses; **anticholinergics** are given for urinary frequency and urgency. Baclofen is useful in treating spasticity; nocturnal spasms can be relieved by diazepam. Diffuse dysesthetic pain responds to carbamazepine or gabapentin.

Complications

As the disease progresses, motor tone increases as does spasticity, bladder dysfunction, and fatigue.

Breakout Point

- The most common demyelinating illness in the CNS
- Manifests as relapsing/remitting symptoms
- Diagnosed clinically in conjunction with MRI findings of periventricular lesions in the white matter

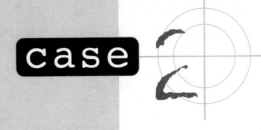

ID/CC A **50-year-old man** presents with **high fever** with chills, severe **headache**, and a **declining mental status**.

HPI He is homeless and had been complaining of cough and fever for the last week. He was found in a stupor.

PE VS: fever (39.5°C); **tachycardia** (HR 130); tachypnea; hypotension (BP 90/60). PE: nonverbal, confused, disoriented, and unable to follow commands; no skin rashes (meningococcal meningitis less likely); nuchal rigidity; **Kernig's and Brudzinski's signs positive**; no cranial nerve palsies; Babinski's sign absent; funduscopy normal.

Labs CBC: leukocytosis (20,000). Normal serum glucose (110 mg/dL). LP: **opening pressure 25 cm water; 2,000 WBCs/μL** (90% PMNs); **glucose 20 mg/dL; protein 170 mg/dL;** CSF Gram stain reveals **gram-positive cocci** in chains. Culture yields *Streptococcus pneumoniae*.

Imaging CT, head: normal.

case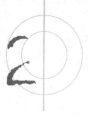

Meningitis—Bacterial

Pathogenesis

Bacteria may infiltrate the meninges via the blood or from adjacent structures; **hematogenous spread is most common** and typically occurs via the upper respiratory tract. Inflammation leads to increased permeability of the blood-brain barrier, which allows fluid and WBCs to enter meninges and can cause edema, increased ICP, and worsened signs of infection. Low glucose in the CSF, high protein, and marked pleocytosis are characteristic of bacterial meningitis; **Gram stain**, which is positive in 80% of cases, is diagnostic. The most common organisms involved are *Haemophilus influenzae, Neisseria meningitidis,* and *S. pneumoniae.*

Epidemiology

S. pneumoniae **is the most common cause of meningitis in adults** and the second most common cause in children older than 6 years. Seventy percent of cases are in children under 2 years old.

Management

Empiric IV ceftriaxone and vancomycin; then narrow the antibiotic spectrum when organism susceptibility results return. In cases of increased ICP, use **steroids.**

Complications

Pneumococcal meningitis has a significant mortality rate and is associated with residual neurologic deficits, seizures, and sepsis. Coma and pneumonia are associated with a poor prognosis. Rapid killing of bacteria may result in inflammation that leads to increased permeability of the blood-brain barrier, edema, and increased ICP.

Breakout Point

- Brudzinski sign: Passive neck flexion in a supine patient resulting in flexion of the knees and hips
- Kernig sign: With the patient lying supine and the hip flexed at 90°, extension of the knee elicits resistance or pain in the lower back or posterior thigh
- CSF findings: neutrophils, low glucose, high protein

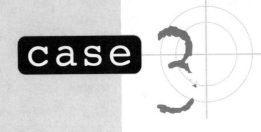

case

ID/CC A **25-year-old woman** presents with **frontal headache, fever,** photophobia, and **neck stiffness** for 2 days.

HPI She had a URI 2 weeks ago. She now also complains of nausea and **vomiting.**

PE VS: fever. PE: alert and oriented; **mild nuchal rigidity; Kernig's and Brudzinski's signs negative;** no focal deficits; funduscopy normal.

Labs CBC: normal. Lytes: normal (serum glucose 125 mg/dL). LP: opening pressure 11 cm water; clear; CSF **glucose 100 mg/dL; 20 WBCs with 90% lymphocytes; mildly elevated protein;** CSF Gram stain reveals no organisms.

Imaging CT, head: normal.

case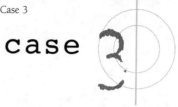

Meningitis—Aseptic

Pathogenesis

Aseptic meningitis is a common, rarely fatal inflamm-ation of the leptomeninges and presents with CSF mononuclear pleocytosis. Enteroviruses, mumps virus, arborvirus, HSV, HIV, and medications (ibupro-fen) are causes of aseptic meningitis.

Epidemiology

Incidence is 1 in 10,000 per year. A specific pathogen is rarely identified.

Management

Treat with bed rest, analgesics, and antipyretics. Full recovery can be expected 5 to 14 days after symptom onset.

Complications

The prognosis is excellent in adults; rare complications in infants include hearing loss and learning disabilities. Hyponatremia may develop as a result of SIADH.

Breakout Point

- Lumbar puncture is contraindicated with increased ICP, sepsis, focal neurological signs, Glasgow coma score <13, infection at the LP site, bleeding disorder, or confident diagnosis of meningococcal infection.
- CSF findings: lymphocytes, normal glucose, high protein

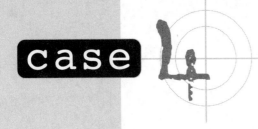

ID/CC   A **23-year-old man,** who immigrated to the United States from **Nigeria** 6 months ago, presents with worsening **headache, neck stiffness,** and difficulty walking for the past 2 weeks.

HPI   For the past month, he has been having **generalized malaise** and **fatigue.** For the past 2 weeks, he has had **weakness** of the **right side.**

PE   VS: fever (101.4°F). PE: **Nuchal rigidity. Kernig's and Brudzinki's signs** are present. Weakness of right face, arm, and leg.

Labs   LP: **opening pressure** is elevated at **35 mmHg.** CSF is clear, with 102 WBCs (lymphocytic predominance), low glucose (30), and high protein (186). AFB smear is negative, **TB PCR is positive.**

Imaging   MRI, brain: meningeal enhancement, large enhancing lesion in the left basal ganglia.

case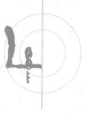

Tuberculous Meningitis

Pathogenesis | **Tuberculous meningitis** usually results from **reactivation** of latent infection with **Mycobacterium tuberculosis**. After primary infection, bacilli seed the meninges of the brain via **hematologic spread** from the respiratory system. These organisms typically remain dormant until a **tubercle ruptures into the subarachnoid space** causing CSF dissemination and subsequent meningitis.

Epidemiology | Approximately one-third of the world's population is infected with TB and about 10% will develop clinical manifestations of the disease. The risk for TB increases in patients with **advanced age, immunosuppression** due to **HIV** or **immunosuppressive therapy,** and history of **alcoholism** or **IV drug use.**

Management | **Multiagent therapy** is the mainstay in the initial therapy, until culture and susceptibility tests results are known. Treatment consists of a combination of **isoniazid, rifampin, pyrazinamide,** and **ethambutol. Corticosteroids** are indicated as adjunctive therapy for severely ill patients with **spinal subarachnoid block, increased ICP,** or **cerebral edema.**

Complications | Hydrocephalus, brain edema, spinal block (blockage of CSF flow anywhere in the spinal canal), and cranial nerve palsies, stroke due to vasculitis, and seizures.

Breakout Point |
- Clinical suspicion is high in HIV, immigrants from developing countries, transplant patients, IV drug use, chronic steroid use, prisoners
- CSF findings: lymphocytes, low glucose, very high protein

case 5

ID/CC A **30-year-old man** complains of moderate **headache**, nausea, **vomiting, fever** with chills, and muscle aches for the past 2 days.

HPI Three days ago, his wife noted that he **started to "forget things."** He has also been unable to name familiar objects such as a radio (ANOMIC APHASIA). His wife has noted **speech difficulty** and episodes of irritable behavior over the past 24 hours. He also has been **smelling nonexistent odors** (OLFACTORY HALLUCINATIONS, indicative of seizure).

PE VS: **fever** (38.4°C); **tachycardia** (HR 120); **tachypnea** (RR 24). PE: mildly confused and disoriented; **mild nuchal rigidity;** speech notable for **paraphasic errors** (e.g., "shoon" instead of "spoon"); patient follows simple (one-step) commands and approximately 50% of complex (three-step) commands; he can draw a clock and bisect lines correctly (tests of nondominant parietal lobe function) and can add and subtract two-digit numbers but cannot perform simple (one-digit) multiplication problems; cranial nerves intact; motor strength 5/5 bilaterally; DTRs 2+ and symmetric throughout; patient withdraws limbs to painful stimuli.

Labs CBC/Lytes: normal. PT/PTT, BUN, and creatinine normal. LFTs: normal. LP: opening pressure of 100 mm water; **protein elevated** (100 mg/dL); **glucose normal;** elevated WBC count with **mononuclear pleocytosis** (100 WBCs/mL); **red cells present** (often a hemorrhagic process); CSF culture negative (positive in HSV-2); **HSV** DNA **PCR** in CSF positive.

Imaging CT, head: bilateral temporal lobe hypodensity.

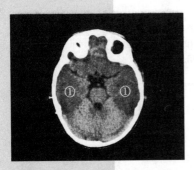

Figure 5-1. CT, head: bilateral temporal lobe hypodensity [1].

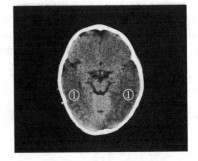

Figure 5-2. MR, brain: **T2 hyperintensity** involving the cortex and white matter in the **temporal lobes.**

9

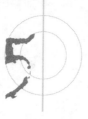

case 5

Herpes Simplex Encephalitis

Pathogenesis

Ninety-five percent of cases of herpes simplex encephalitis are due to **HSV type 1**. The ports of entry are the oropharyngeal mucosa, conjunctiva, or broken skin; the virus **replicates locally and enters the sensory nerves.** From the sensory nerves, the virus is transported to the sensory nerve ganglia, where it remains latent. The factors that induce activation of the latent virus and the mechanism by which the virus targets the temporal lobes are not well understood. Untreated patients rapidly deteriorate to coma and death in 70% of cases.

Epidemiology

HSV encephalitis is the most common identified cause of acute sporadic viral encephalitis. HSV-1 encephalitis occurs in all age groups, in both sexes, and during all seasons.

Management

Treat with **IV acyclovir.** Mannitol and corticosteroids relieve cerebral edema. Phenytoin is used to treat seizures. Repeat LP after treatment to ensure that there is no residual infection.

Complications

Persistent seizures, recurrent lymphocytic meningitis, and neurologic deficits. Amnesia is a prominent residual symptom.

Breakout Point

- MRI Brain shows hypodensity in inferomedial temporal and frontal lobes
- CSF findings: lymphocytes, normal glucose, high protein, many RBC

case 6

ID/CC An **8-year-old boy** presents with **"jerking"** movements.

HPI The boy has no significant medical history and does not have a regular pediatrician. His mother cannot remember if his vaccinations are up to date. He had **measles at 10 months of age** but has developed normally. In the last month, his grades at school have worsened considerably. Two days ago, his mother noted the onset of continuous "jerking" movements.

PE VS: normal. PE: **lethargic** but able to cooperate; neck supple; cranial nerves intact; motor tone exceptional given continuous **myoclonic movements** involving all four extremities; DTRs 2+ and symmetric throughout; finger-to-nose exam reveals mild **dysmetria**; ataxic gait; sensation intact to pinprick in all four extremities.

Labs CBC: normal. EEG: **burst suppression**. LP: normal opening pressure; normal protein and glucose with no white cells; CSF antibody titer **elevated** for **measles-specific antibodies.** No organisms on Gram stain; **elevated oligoclonal bands** (indicative of inflammatory process).

Imaging CT, head: cerebral edema and diffuse hypodense signal in white matter bilaterally.

case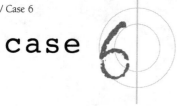

Subacute Sclerosing Panencephalitis

Pathogenesis

Subacute sclerosing panencephalitis (SSPE) occurs due to **accumulation of defective measles virus in neurons** and a subsequent inappropriate immune response to accumulated viral nucleic acid and proteins. The measles virus may also reactivate, usually 2 to 10 years after the original viral attack. SSPE is characterized by **three clinical stages:** stage I is marked by behavioral and cognitive decline; stage II by motor dysfunction (spasticity, weakness) and often myoclonic jerks and seizures; and stage III by stupor, coma, and autonomic failure (loss of thermoregulation). Death occurs 1 to 3 years after onset of symptoms.

Epidemiology

Fewer than 10 cases per year in the United States with higher incidence in the Middle East and India. Average age of onset is 6 to 8 years; the median interval between acute measles infection and SSPE is 8 years. **Males** are affected three times more often than females. Large-scale measles vaccination programs have resulted in a twentyfold decrease in the risk of SSPE.

Management

Prevention by measles vaccination; **supportive care.** Antiepileptic treatment if seizures occur. Immunomodulators (e.g., interferon) and antivirals (e.g., ribavirin).

Complications

Seizures, autonomic failure, coma, and death.

Breakout Point

- Occurs years after an attack of measles
- Demyelinating, immune-mediated destruction of white matter
- Presents as seizures, myoclonic jerks, stupor, death

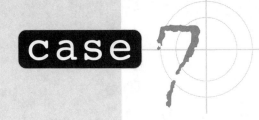

case 7

ID/CC A **62-year-old woman** with a history of **untreated venereal disease** complains of sudden electric-like **lancinating pain** in both legs and **"stumbling"** whenever she turns quickly.

HPI Three months ago, she started experiencing intermittent, brief, sharp stabbing pains in both legs, followed by **gait unsteadiness,** particularly at night. She also complains of **urinary incontinence.**

PE VS: normal. PE: **discrepancy in pupillary size** (ANISOCORIA); involved pupil **does not react to light but constricts on accommodation** (ARGYLL-ROBERTSON PUPIL). Sensory exam shows **decreased vibration and joint position sense** in both legs to the level of the knees, with mild loss of sensation to pinprick and temperature. Strength is full in her extremities. **Reflexes are absent** in the legs and Babinski sign is absent. Her gait is slightly **wide-based,** and she cannot walk tandem. The **Romberg sign is present.**

Labs CBC/Lytes: normal. **RPR** was positive (titer of 1:128) and **FTA-ABS** was also positive. LP: **lymphocytic pleocytosis** (15 lymphocytes) and **protein elevated** (65 mg/dL). CSF **VDRL** was also positive.

Imaging MRI, spine: degeneration of the posterior column in the sacral and thoracic cord.

case 7

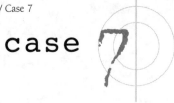

Tabes Dorsalis

Pathogenesis

Tabes dorsalis generally occurs 10 to 20 years after untreated primary infection by the spirochete *Treponema pallidum.* Tabes dorsalis is a form of **teritiary neurosyphilis,** characterized by progressive **degeneration of the posterior columns and dorsal root ganglia,** due to persistent infection. Ataxia results from destruction of the **proprioceptive** pathways, while damage to the **small sensory fibers** cause **pain** in the limbs and the viscera. Patients also have **bladder hypotonia** from sacral root involvement causing **overflow incontinence.**

Epidemiology

There was a rise in the incidence of neurosyphilis in the 1990s due to the increasing incidence of HIV/AIDS infections.

Management

IV penicillin G. Successful treatment is demonstrated by follow up CSF studies at 6 months with normal count and decreasing protein content.

Complications

Charcot joints, perforating foot ulcers, weakness and atrophy if the motor roots are involved, fecal incontinence, visual impairment, and deafness.

Breakout Point

- Argyll Robertson pupil (does not constrict to light but does constrict to accommodation)
- Degeneration of the posterior columns
- Treated with IV penicillin G

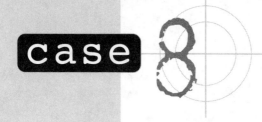

ID/CC A **33-year-old right-handed man** with a history of **HIV** infection presents with 3 weeks of **slurred speech** and **progressive left-sided weakness.**

HPI He has not been compliant with his HIV treatment and stopped taking his antiretroviral medications more than 6 months ago. He was treated for **PCP pneumonia** and **oral thrush** 2 months ago. For the past 3 weeks, he has been slurring his speech, slow to respond, and has been having progressive left-sided weakness to the point where he cannot walk without assistance.

PE VS: normal. PE: Very thin man. Oriented and answers questions correctly but is extremely slow with his responses. Speech is slow and **dysarthric.** Flattening of the left-nasolabial fold and significant weakness of the left arm and leg. **Hyperreflexia** of the left side with five beats of **sustained clonus** at the left ankle.

Labs CBC: **low CD4 count** (46). LP: normal opening pressure, normal cell count, glucose, and protein. **CSF PCR** for **JC virus** is **positive.**

Imaging MRI, brain: large confluent areas of T2 hyperintensities in the subcortical white matter bilaterally.

case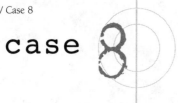

Progressive Multifocal Leukodystrophy

Pathogenesis

Progressive multifocal leukodystrophy (PML) results from reactivation of a **papovavirus** called **JC virus.** The virus is typically present in the healthy population and resides dormant in the kidneys and lungs, with 90% of individuals showing antibodies to the virus. In **immunocompromised** patients, the virus gains access to the CNS via **hematogenous spread** and selectively infects the **oligodendrocytes,** causing widespread **demyelination.** The disorder usually runs a subacute course of progressive **subcortical dementia** and ultimately **death within 6 months.**

Epidemiology

Extremely rare in immunocompetent individuals. PML occurred in approximately 4% of patients with AIDS, but use of antiretroviral therapy has reduced the incidence.

Management

No definitive therapy for PML. Antiviral agents such as cytarabine (ARA-C), cidofovir, and HAART may halt progression, but no consistent success has been demonstrated.

Complications

Aspiration pneumonia, side effects from drug therapies.

Breakout Point

- Demyelinating disease caused by JC virus infection
- Occurs in immunocompromised patients (HIV)
- Death in 6 months

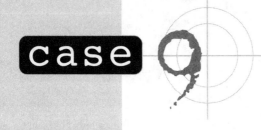
ID/CC A **50-year-old woman** presents with sudden-onset left-sided **facial weakness, hearing loss,** and **ear pain** of 2 days' duration.

HPI She also has left-sided **throat pain,** tinnitus, vertigo, and **altered taste sensation.** She recently underwent radiation treatment for an unidentified lymphoma (immune-compromised state).

PE **Vesicular rash** on left external ear (herpes zoster); **sensorineural hearing loss** on left side; taste absent on left anterior third of tongue; **left-sided peripheral facial palsy.**

Labs CBC: lymphocytosis. LP: **elevated protein** in CSF. **Tzanck smear of vesicles positive.**

Imaging CT, head: no intracranial lesions or hemorrhage.

case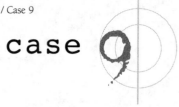

Ramsay Hunt Syndrome

Pathogenesis

Ramsay Hunt syndrome, or herpes zoster oticus, is an acute facial paralysis that occurs with herpetic blisters of the skin of the ear canal or auricle. Herpes zoster reactivation is promoted by radiation and immune compromise, including that associated with lympho-proliferative disorders, HIV, and cytotoxic chemo-therapy. The virus remains dormant in nerve roots and ganglia. Herpes zoster reactivation is also called **shingles;** when it involves the **seventh and eighth cranial nerves,** it is designated Ramsay Hunt syndrome.

Epidemiology

The incidence in children is low; in adults, it is appro-ximately 2.5 per 1,000 per year.

Management

Acyclovir reduces the duration of the vesicular rash and diminishes the likelihood of postherpetic neuralgia. **Corticosteroids** also may be used as adjuvant therapy to shorten the duration and reduce the chance of post-herpetic neuralgia.

Complications

Hearing loss, reactivation of virus, meningoencephalitis in immunocompromised patients.

Breakout Point

- Develops after HSV infection or reactivation
- Herpes vesicles in ear canal, affecting cranial nerves
- Presents with facial paresis, tinnitus, vertigo, and ipsilateral hearing loss

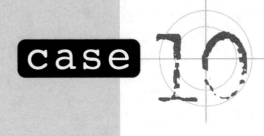

case 10

ID/CC A **4-year-old girl** who was **born prematurely** presents with **difficulty walking.**

HPI The child was born after a difficult delivery, at 28 weeks. Almost all developmental milestones (especially motor) were delayed and she has learned to walk only within the past year. Her parents have noted that her **gait is clumsy and stiff** (SPASTIC GAIT). She also has abnormal, **abrupt, jerky movements of her limbs** (CHOREA) and sometimes **slow, writhing, continuous movements** (ATHETOSIS).

PE Motor strength 4/5 in both lower extremities and 5/5 in both upper extremities; **motor tone increased** in lower extremities but normal in upper extremities; DTRs 3+ bilaterally in lower extremities and 2+ bilaterally in upper extremities; **Moro's and asymmetric tonic neck reflexes persist.**

Labs None.

Imaging MR, brain: **periventricular white matter disease.**

case 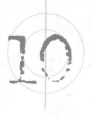 10

Cerebral Palsy

Pathogenesis | Cerebral palsy is a motor deficit of **unknown etiology** due to a nonprogressive lesion in the immature brain. The pathology may occur at any stage of brain development. Premature newborns may suffer from periventricular hemorrhage affecting the white matter, which primarily carries that portion of the corticospinal tract that is responsible for leg movement.

Epidemiology | Cerebral palsy is associated with **cerebral anoxia** at birth, **prematurity, trauma, embryologic malformations,** and **infection.**

Management | Initiate **physical and occupational therapy** at birth. Orthotic devices may be necessary if ambulation is significantly affected. Treat associated problems such as seizures and learning disabilities.

Complications | Complications depend on the severity of cerebral palsy. If mobility is severely limited, patients may suffer from pneumonia, UTIs, and decubitus ulcers. Associated problems include epilepsy, mental retardation, behavioral problems, and learning disabilities.

Breakout Point

- Movement disorder caused by defects or lesions of the immature brain
- Associated with prenatal factors in 75% of cases

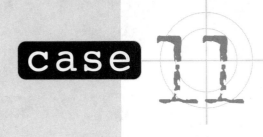

case 11

ID/CC A **19-year-old woman** presents with **decreasing performance in college** and an **abnormal eye exam.**

HPI The patient's mother states her daughter has been **clumsy** with her hands, **trips** occasionally while walking, and sometimes **slurs her speech.** Her personality has also been changing.

PE VS: normal. PE: mask-like facies; drooling; **mild RUQ tenderness**; mildly decreased strength throughout; asymmetric **resting tremor**; slit-lamp eye exam reveals **golden crescent discoloration** around the perimeter of the cornea (KAYSER-FLEISCHER RING).

Labs CBC/Lytes: normal. LFTs: elevated liver transaminases and total bilirubin. **Low serum ceruloplasmin. Increased urinary copper excretion.** Liver biopsy reveals fatty infiltration, portal inflammation, and fibrosis with increased **copper.**

Imaging MRI, brain: copper deposition in the lenticular nuclei and the caudate nuclei.

case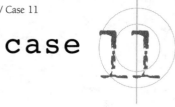

Wilson's Disease

Pathogenesis	Wilson's disease (**hepatolenticular degeneration**) is an autosomal recessive disease that is inherited when two copies of the gene for the ATP7B protein (a membrane based ATP-dependent copper transporter) are mutated and nonfunctional. Lack of proper copper trafficking in the cell leads to **accumulation of copper** (which is usually eliminated through the biliary system) and **decreased ceruloplasmin** formation (the major carrier of copper in the blood). Increased copper stores in the body are deposited in the **liver, brain, and eyes.** The diagnosis is often made during childhood to young adulthood, most commonly with **hepatitis** as the presenting symptom, which may lead to **cirrhosis.** The brain is primarily affected in the **basal ganglia** (especially in the putamen). **Kayser-Fleischer rings** are caused by copper deposition in the cornea (Descemet's membrane).
Epidemiology	Wilson's disease is **rare,** affecting 1 in 30,000 people. 4:1 **female** predominance.
Management	**D-Penicillamine:** causes copper chelation and urinary excretion (many side effects). Trientine: copper chelation with fewer side effects but less efficacious than D-Penicillamine in some patients; oral zinc: binds copper in the gut and causes fecal excretion; low copper diet. Liver transplantation.
Complications	Liver cancer, fulminant decompensated liver failure. Fatal if untreated (average age of death is 30 years).
Breakout Point	• Autosomal recessive inheritance • Increased copper, decreased ceruloplasmin • Triad of cirrhosis, neurologic manifestations, and Kayser-Fleischer ring

■ TABLE 11-1 WILSON'S DISEASE CLINICAL PRESENTATIONS

Neuropsychiatric	Tremor, clumsiness, rigidity, speech slurring, drooling, uncontrollable grinning (risus sardonicus), dyskinesia, personality changes
Hepatic	Chronic hepatitis, liver function tests abnormalities, portal hypertension
Ophthalmologic	Kayser-Fleischer ring

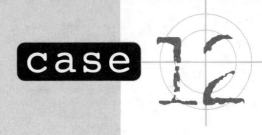

case **12**

ID/CC	A **31-year-old woman** presents with **headaches, nausea, and vomiting** of 2 months' duration.
HPI	The headaches have slowly increased in severity over the past month. She denies any change in vision or motor weakness. Her **mother died of cancer** at the age of 28.
PE	VS: normal. PE: speech appropriate; mild papilledema in right disk; left disk not well visualized secondary to **enlarged globular blood vessel** (HAMARTOMA); finger-to-nose exam significant for mild **dysmetria;** gait slightly **wide-based;** tandem gait severely impaired; sensory exam intact.
Labs	CBC: **polycythemia** (due to ectopic erythropoietin production by hemangioblastoma).
Imaging	CT, brain: large, low-density, **cystic-appearing mass in the midline of the cerebellum.** CT, abdomen: multiple **bilateral renal cysts.**

case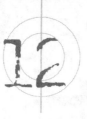

Von Hippel–Lindau Disease

Pathogenesis
: Von Hippel–Lindau disease is an **autosomal dominant** disease hallmarked by development of **hemangioblastomas** in the **retina** and **cerebellum**, **pheochromocytomas**, and multiple **cysts** of the pancreas and **kidneys**. Within the same family, all gradations of the syndrome may be found. The gene locus for von Hippel–Lindau disease has been mapped to **chromosome 3p.**

Epidemiology
: Becomes symptomatic during adult life and has an **autosomal-dominant** pattern of inheritance.

Management
: **Surgical excision** of hemangioblastomas (surgical approach aided by cerebral angiogram). Annual ophthalmologic exams to screen for **retinal hemangioblastoma.**

Complications
: Retinal hemangioblastoma, recurrence of hemangioblastoma, adrenal abnormalities (pheochromocytoma, adrenal medulla cyst, adrenal cortical hyperplasia), and renal carcinoma.

Breakout Point

- Autosomal dominant inheritance
- Presents with hemangioblastomas of the retina, cerebellum, brainstem, spinal cord
- Presents with cysts in pancreas and kidneys, pheochromocytomas
- Increased incidence of renal cell carcinoma

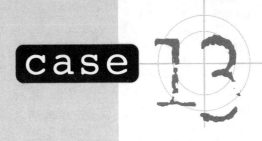

case 13

ID/CC A **10-year-old boy** is seen by a neurologist because of **progressive difficulty walking** and **diminution of vision**.

HPI The patient has a **right foot deformity** (pes cavus). After suffering two episodes of syncope, he presented to a cardiologist and was diagnosed with **hypertrophic cardiomyopathy**. His parents give a history of **consanguineous marriage; an uncle**, who had a similar illness, **died of cardiac complications**.

PE VS: normal. PE: wide-based **ataxia**; nystagmus; dysarthria; **areflexia** in lower extremities; **Babinski sign present; joint position sense** and vibratory sense **lost in lower limbs;** pain and temperature sensations intact; intellect normal; spastic weakness in lower extremities with 4+ strength in select muscle groups in upper extremities; distal wasting apparent, especially in upper extremities; optic atrophy.

Labs Elevated blood glucose (200 mg/dL); indicative of overt **diabetes mellitus**.

Imaging None.

case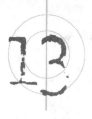

Friedreich's Ataxia

Pathogenesis

Friedreich's ataxia exhibits an **autosomal-recessive inheritance**; the gene locus has been mapped to chromosome 9, which holds excessive trinucleotide DNA repeats of the GAA (guanine adenine adenine) sequence. Classically, **three long tracts degenerate:** the pyramidal, dorsal, and spinocerebellar. Accompanying abnormalities include **cardiomyopathy,** skeletal abnormalities, optic atrophy, and an increased incidence of diabetes mellitus.

Epidemiology

Roughly 50% of patients with hereditary ataxia have Friedreich's ataxia. Presents in children and involves ataxia with progressive involvement of all the extremities. The mean age of death is in the mid-40s.

Management

No specific treatment is available. Diabetes mellitus, when diagnosed, requires management. Cardiomyopathy often results in arrhythmias that need treatment. Physical therapy and walking aids.

Complications

Cardiomyopathy is often the cause of death, usually before age 40. Progressive neurologic decompensation results in loss of ambulation within 5 years after the onset of symptoms.

Breakout Point

- Autosomal recessive inheritance
- Presents with progressive gait and truncal ataxia, dysarthria, areflexia in the lower extremities, and extensor plantar responses (positive Babinski sign)
- Trinucleotide repeat disorder

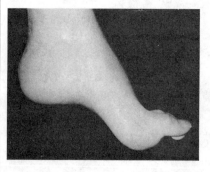

Figure 13-1. Typical pes cavus foot deformity seen in Friedreich's ataxia.

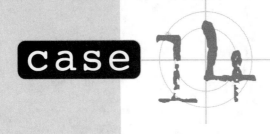

ID/CC A **57-year-old right-handed woman** presents with a **closed right eye.**

HPI She has HTN and DM. She complains of intermittent right-sided headache, **double vision,** and a **droopy eyelid** for the past week. She woke up this morning and found her right eye completely shut. She was unable to voluntarily open it.

PE VS: hypertensive. PE: Her right eyelid is closed. When the right eyelid is passively lifted, the right eye **deviates down and out,** and **the pupil is fixed and dilated** at 6 mm. She is able to abduct and intort the right eye. The disc is normal bilaterally. The left pupil and eye movements are normal. The rest of her examination is normal.

Labs Normal.

Imaging Cerebral angiogram.

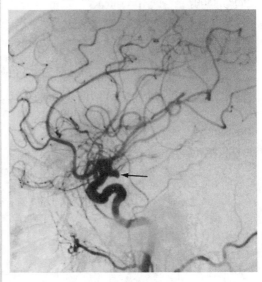

Figure 14-1. Cerebral angiogram: aneurysm (arrow) of the posterior communicating artery.

CRANIAL NERVE

case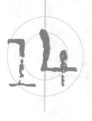

Oculomotor Nerve Palsy

Pathogenesis

This third CN palsy was caused by a cerebral aneurysm of the posterior communicating artery. Aneurysms are most commonly congenital. They develop due to weakness of the vessel wall (especially near branching points) and may take a **saccular or fusiform** shape. Saccular aneurysms are most commonly found around the **Circle of Willis** and may be multiple in 20% of patients. They can be associated with many conditions such as polycystic kidney disease, Marfan syndrome, and coarctation of the aorta. An aneurysm of the posterior communicating artery causes compression of CN III, resulting in a fixed and dilated pupil, ptosis, and the eye sits down and out, due to weakness of all of the eye muscles, except the superior oblique (innervated by the CN IV), and the lateral rectus (innervated by the CN VI).

Epidemiology

The prevalence of intracranial aneurysms ranges between 1% and 6% of adults.

Management

Early treatment to **secure the aneurysm** by surgical clipping or by coiling is the best treatment option, especially for those with good baseline function.

Complications

Subarachnoid hemorrhage, focal neurologic deficits due to compression of nearby structures due to expansion of aneurysm.

Breakout Point

- Surgical third nerve palsy: pupil fixed and dilated, which constitutes a surgical emergency
- Medical third nerve palsy: pupil-sparing palsy, frequently associated with diabetes mellitus

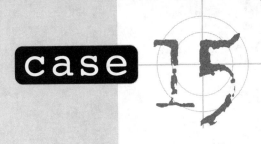

case 15

ID/CC A **52-year-old woman** complains of episodes of severe **pain in the right cheek** with muscle spasm over the past year.

HPI The pain is **electric in character** and **occurs while she is brushing her teeth.** Each episode lasts <2 minutes. At first, the episodes occurred daily for 3 to 4 days and then disappeared for 2 months. For the past 3 weeks, volleys of attacks have occurred everyday and are sometimes triggered by face washing, chewing, or a light breeze.

PE VS: normal. PE: mild touch in **right V2** (maxillary subdivision of trigeminal) **distribution** reproduces the painful episode; remainder of neurologic exam normal.

Labs ESR: normal.

Imaging MR, brain: normal.

case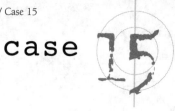

Trigeminal Neuralgia

Pathogenesis

Trigeminal neuralgia is usually **idiopathic,** but may be caused by a meningioma that compresses the gasserian ganglion, by a schwannoma of the nerve, by malignant infiltration of the skull base, or by herpes zoster infection. V2 or V3 distributions are more commonly affected than V1. The typical course is relapsing/remitting over several years.

Epidemiology

Most idiopathic cases begin after age 50. Twice as common in females as in males. Ninety percent of patients are **older than 40 years.**

Management

Carbamazepine, gabapentin, **phenytoin,** or baclofen. If medical treatment fails, then multiple **surgical treatments** are available, including alcohol block of the affected branch of the trigeminal nerve as well as percutaneous thermocoagulation of the trigeminal nerve sensory root (the procedure of choice in the elderly).

Breakout Point

- Also called tic douloureux
- Lancinating facial pain in V2, V3 territory
- Presents as extreme pain with movement, eating, air drafts, light touch

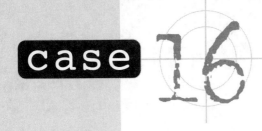

case 16

ID/CC   A **30-year-old woman** presents with new-onset right-sided **facial weakness** and **drooping of the right side of the mouth.**

HPI   She complains of a sore right eye (due to drying of the cornea). She also becomes irritated on hearing even minor noises, complaining that they are "too loud" (HYPERACUSIS).

PE   Alert and oriented ×3; funduscopy normal; right-sided **paralysis of upper and lower face** such that eye cannot be closed tightly (or can easily be opened by physician); eyeball turns up on attempted closure (BELL'S PHENOMENON); she is **unable to raise right eyebrow** (LOWER MOTOR NEURON RIGHT FACIAL PALSY); corner of mouth droops and **nasolabial fold** is **decreased;** voluntary and involuntary movements of mouth are paralyzed on right side (lips are drawn to opposite side); examination of right ear normal (to rule out herpetic Ramsay Hunt syndrome); no other CN palsy found; no other neurologic deficit.

Labs   None.

Imaging   MR, brain (with gadolinium): no intracranial lesions; shows facial nerve enhancement. CT, head: no intracranial lesions or hemorrhage.

CRANIAL NERVE

case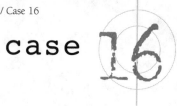

Bell's Palsy

Pathogenesis	Bell's palsy is an abrupt, unilateral, peripheral facial paresis, and (as a diagnosis of exclusion) it is, by definition, **idiopathic**. It may have a viral etiology and is popularly thought to result from compression of an inflamed facial nerve as it courses through the facial canal of the temporal bone. Approximately 80% of patients recover fully.
Epidemiology	The **most common form of facial paralysis.**
Management	Current guidelines support use of **glucocorticoids**. Antiviral therapy is commonly used. Because HSV is the most widely accepted cause of Bell's palsy, treat with **acyclovir. Protect the eye** with artificial tears and taping the eye shut at night.
Complications	Chronic paralysis in a minority of cases.
Breakout Point	

- Sudden lower motor neuron paralysis of facial nerve
- Associated with hyperacusis or impaired taste
- More common in pregnant women or diabetics

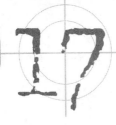

ID/CC A **75-year-old right-handed woman** was brought in by her family when they noticed that she had become increasingly **forgetful**.

HPI She has been having **difficulty remembering people's names, dates** (such as her children's birthdays), missed several medical appointments, and **lost her way in a familiar surrounding** (loss of visual-spatial abilities).

PE She is well-groomed and very polite. She could register three objects but could not recall any of them. She had difficulty with naming (ANOMIA) and used incorrect words (PARAPHASIC ERRORS). Generating a list of animals was very difficult. She made errors with additions and subtractions and could not accurately copy inter-secting pentagons (CONSTRUCTIONAL APRAXIA).

Labs CBC, BMP, LFTs, TFTs, and B$_{12}$ level were all normal. RPR was nonreactive.

Imaging CT, head: nonspecific cerebral atrophy and widened third ventricle. MRI, brain: mild diffuse atrophy of the temporal and parietal lobes and localized atrophy at the hippocampus. Also, widened third ventricle.

Pathology There are two hallmark features on histopathology, including **neurofibrillary tangles** and **neuritic amyloid plaques**, which are most prominent in the **hippocampal region**.

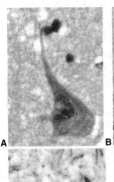
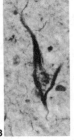
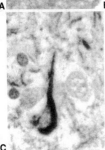

Figure 17-1. Neuritic plaques with central amyloid cores by three methods of staining.

case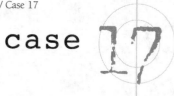

Alzheimer's Disease

Pathogenesis

Alzheimer's disease (AD) is a neurodegenerative disorder causing progressive cognitive decline. It is usually **sporadic,** but a **genetic** basis has been identified in certain families. The Apo-E4 allele and mutations in **presenilin 1, presenilin 2, amyloid precursor protein genes,** have all been associated with familial AD and increased susceptibility to AD. Also, expression of tau protein is increased in neurons that eventually develop neurofibrillary tangles. Neurochemically, the acetylcholine-synthesizing enzyme **choline acetyltransferase** (chAT) is markedly **depleted** in the cerebral cortex and hippocampus. A deficiency in cholinergic transmission, for example, loss of cholinergic projections to the nucleus basalis of Meynert, has been hypothesized as correlative to the severity of memory loss.

Epidemiology

AD is the most common cause of dementia. Prevalence increases with age, especially >65 years. Men and women are equally affected. Patients with **Down Syndrome** are more likely to have early onset AD. Approximately 1 to 4% of those from age 65 to age 70 are affected, and 22% or more are in the age group of 85 to 90.

Management

No available treatment that can reverse or arrest disease progression. **Acetylcholinesterase inhibitors** such as **donepezil, rivastigmine, and galantamine** preserve acetylcholine by inactivating its metabolic enzyme. They have been used for symptomatic treatment in mild and moderate stages of the disease. Given with donepezil, **memantine** (an NMDA receptor antagonist) may block toxic glutamine excitation, another approach to improving memory.

Complications

Wandering behavior may compromise safety.

Breakout Point

- Most common cause of dementia
- Hallmark pathologic features: neurofibrillary tangles and amyloid plaques.

case 18

ID/CC An **81-year-old right-handed man** with a history of insulin-dependent diabetes mellitus (IDDM) and **hypertension** presents with gradually progressing confusion over the past several years.

HPI He has had **two strokes** with residual left hemiparesis; he was brought to the hospital by his wife due to **increasing confusion** and **angry outbursts.** He has forgotten important appointments, repeatedly **asks the same questions,** and **forgets names** (all due to memory impairment). He has also become irritable, easily frustrated, and suspicious and demanding of his wife (all due to behavioral impairment). For the past 2 years, he has not driven a car because he becomes confused at intersections. He has recently been **getting lost** when he takes walks (due to visual and spatial disorientation).

PE VS: **hypertension** (BP 150/90). PE: pleasant and alert; **oriented to person only;** speech fluent; **cannot recall current president or recent news events,** and **cannot perform mathematical calculations** (serial sevens, simple addition and subtraction); mild left facial droop; 4/5 strength in left upper and lower extremities with mild increase in tone; 5/5 strength in right upper and lower extremities; DTRs 3+ in left upper and lower extremities and 2+ in right upper and lower extremities; **positive snout and palmar-mental reflexes** (PRIMITIVE REFLEXES); **Babinski's sign present bilaterally** (sign of global hemispheric dysfunction); withdraws to pain in all four extremities; finger-to-nose intact bilaterally.

Labs CBC: normal. Serum VDRL, TFTs, B_{12}, and folate levels normal. EEG: moderate to marked generalized slowing; no epileptiform activity.

Imaging CT, head: diffuse **periventricular hypodensity;** small old ischemic infarcts; no hemorrhage; no mass.

case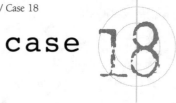

Vascular Dementia

Pathogenesis

Vascular dementia is an accumulation of defects from **multiple, bilateral cerebral infarcts.** Patients with previous cerebral insults will have reduced cerebral reserve and are more vulnerable to confusion from minor insults. Dementia can be classified as cortical or subcortical. **Cortical** causes include primary degenerative dementias such as Alzheimer's, Pick's disease, Creutzfeldt–Jakob disease, multi-infarct dementia, and dementias due to other causes such as normal pressure hydrocephalus, mass lesions, drugs, and HIV. **Subcortical** dementias include Parkinson's and Huntington's dementia.

Epidemiology

Causes 15 to 30% of all dementias; typically occurs in **patients older than 50 years** with a **history of generalized atherosclerotic disease. Men** are affected more often than women.

Management

Aggressive **control of hypertension,** hyperlipidemia, and diabetes to prevent further decline. **Neuroleptics** may be administered for control of aggressive behavior.

Complications

Urinary incontinence, seizure disorder (infarcted regions can serve as a seizure focus), and dysphagia resulting in aspiration pneumonia.

Breakout Point

- Risk factors: hypertension, smoking, hypercholesterolemia, diabetes, coronary artery disease, stroke
- Sudden, distinct, step-wise neurologic deterioration
- Etiology is multiple infarcts

ID/CC   A **54-year-old man** was brought the emergency room after 1 week of **confusion and lethargy.**

HPI   He has a history of **chronic alcohol abuse** and **poor eating habits.**

PE   VS: mild hypothermia and hypotensive. PE: **lethargic,** intermittently opens his eyes briefly to commands. **Not oriented** to place or date. Eye exam: normally reactive pupils, **endgaze nystagmus** on lateral gaze bilaterally, lack of abduction in both eyes (L > R), mild restriction of upward gaze. Wide-based, short-stepped gait. After administration of intravenous **thiamine,** his level of alertness and eye movements return to normal within hours. Memory testing reveals that he has no short-term memory (RETROGRADE AMNESIA), while long-term memory is relatively preserved. He denies any memory problems and **confabulates** to explain events that occurred in the hospital (ANTEROGRADE AMNESIA).

Labs   CBC: macrocytic anemia.

Imaging   CT, brain: diffuse cerebral atrophy.

case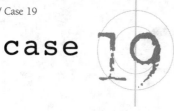

Wernicke-Korsakoff Syndrome

Pathogenesis

Caused by **thiamine (vitamin B₁) deficiency, Wernicke-Korsakoff syndrome** is a two-stage syndrome most frequently seen in **alcoholics** and **severely malnourished** patients. Thiamine is a cofactor involved in glucose metabolism; deficiency causes decreased cerebral glucose utilization. Wernicke's syndrome is characterized by a **triad of acute mental confusion, ophthalmoplegia, and gait ataxia,** due to lesions of the CN nuclei of III and VI. Vestibular dysfunction and involvement of the superior cerebellar vermis are responsible for truncal ataxia. Wernicke's encephalopathy can progress to **Korsakoff's syndrome,** as the ocular and encephalopathic features subside. In Korsakoff's syndrome, memory is impaired out of proportion to other cognitive deficits, and patients are typically unaware of their memory deficit. Pathological studies of Wernicke-Korsakoff syndrome reveal changes in the thalamus, the hypothalamus, the mammillary bodies, the midbrain (periaqueductal areas), the pons and medulla, and the cerebellar vermis.

Epidemiology

The frequency of Wernicke's encephalopathy is estimated at 0.8 to 2.8%, however, clinical recognition of the syndrome is much lower due to underdiagnosis. The mortality rate is 10 to 20%.

Management

IV thiamine as early as possible is the mainstay of therapy, followed daily thiamine 100mg IV or IM. Administer thiamine **before IV glucose** to prevent precipitating or worsening of this condition.

Complications

Persistent ocular deficits, gait ataxia, and memory disturbances.

Breakout Point

- Wernicke's encephalopathy: triad of confusion, ataxia, ophthalmoplegia (CN VI)
- Korsakoff psychosis: anterograde and retrograde amnesia, confabulation

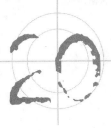
ID/CC A **72-year-old man** presents with **memory loss, gait difficulty,** and **urinary incontinence.**

HPI He was brought to the physician's office by his wife, who states that over the past year he has become increasingly forgetful. She adds that he has also wet his pants and their bed on several occasions (URINARY INCONTINENCE). For the past 6 months, the patient has fallen on numerous occasions and has had difficulty walking in his own home. He has a history of hypertension.

PE VS: normal. PE: no speech defects; impaired short-term memory; unable to demonstrate how to comb his hair (APRAXIA); motor strength 5/5 bilaterally throughout; DTRs 2+; bradykinetic, broad-based gait characterized by short steps; patient can walk only 10 feet before having to sit down.

Labs Serum B_{12}, folate, and TSH normal; VDRL negative. LP: **opening pressure of 90 mm H_2O;** normal glucose and protein; no nucleated cells. After 40 mL of CSF was removed, gait improved.

Imaging CT, head: **enlarged lateral ventricles;** periventricular white matter disease consistent with small-vessel ischemia; no mass, hemorrhage, cortical atrophy, or midline shift.

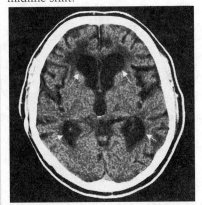

Figure 20-1. CT, head: **enlarged lateral ventricles** with comparatively normal sulci; periventricular white matter disease consistent with small-vessel ischemia; no mass, hemorrhage, cortical atrophy, or midline shift.

DEMENTIA

39

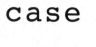 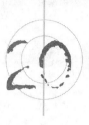

Normal Pressure Hydrocephalus

Pathogenesis

The etiology of normal pressure hydrocephalus is not known; it is likely due to decreased absorption of CSF across the arachnoid villi.

Management

Large-volume LP often results in transient improvement. Approximately 30 to 50% of patients improve following placement of a **ventricular shunt.**

Breakout Point

> 3 Ws of NPH
> **W**obbly (abnormal gait)
> **W**et (urinary incontinence)
> **W**acky (dementia, memory impairment)

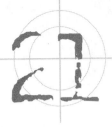

case 21

ID/CC	A **64-year-old woman** was brought into clinic by her daughter because of **visual hallucinations.**
HPI	The patient is adamant that she saw a man climb into her apartment through the window and walk out of her house through the front door. Her daughter, who was with her, did not see anyone and adds that the patient has been making running and punching motions while fast asleep. Low-dose **Haldol** was prescribed for these hallucinations. Unfortunately, the patient developed severe **parkinsonism,** with rigidity, bradykinesia, and a shuffling gait. When the Haldol was stopped, she returned to baseline.
PE	She has slight rigidity in her extremities and is slow in all of her movements. Her short-term memory is intact. The rest of the neurologic examination is unremarkable, and she had no resting tremor.
Labs	CBC, BMP, LFTs, TSH, and B_{12} level are all normal. RPR is nonreactive.
Imaging	PET, brain: occipital lobe hypometabolism.

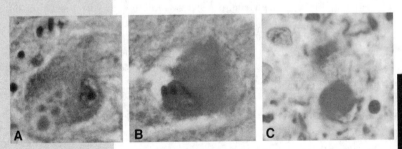

Figure 21-1. Lewy bodies (round intracytoplasmic inclusions) in the substantia nigra neurons (A) and cortical neurons (B and C) are aggregates of α-synuclein, and antibodies to this protein facilitate staining.

case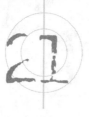

Dementia with Lewy Bodies

Pathogenesis

Dementia with Lewy bodies (DLB) is characterized by **cognitive decline, fluctuations in level of alertness,** and **parkinsonian features** (rigidity and bradykinesia). Although DLB shares many histopathological features with Alzheimer's disease, early **memory impairment is not a prominent feature,** in contrast. Another distinguishing feature of DLB is **detailed and vivid visual hallucinations,** associated with Lewy bodies in the temporal lobes. Lewy bodies also may be found in the cerebral cortex, limbic regions, and brainstem; the concentration of Lewy bodies corresponds to the severity of dementia. About half of patients with DLB develop **REM sleep behavior disorder,** where normal REM-induced sleep paralysis is disrupted by motions, and patients appear to act out their dreams. Although tempting to treat hallucinations with dopamine-blocking antipsychotics, **extrapyramidal side effects** may produce akinesia and board-like rigidity.

Epidemiology

Based on autopsy studies, DLB constitute 20% of dementias. Although DLB, Alzheimer's disease, and Parkinson's disease are considered to be separate entities, there is significant overlap in clinical and pathologic features.

Management

Acetylcholine esterase inhibitors may be useful for mental status symptoms and hallucinations. **Dopaminergic agents** such as L-dopa may minimally benefit parkinsonian symptoms. However, visual hallucinations may worsen, and patients are less responsive than those diagnosed with Parkinson's disease. Long-acting **benzodiazepines,** e.g., clonazepam, for REM sleep behavior disorder.

Complications

Falls due to gait instability, pneumonia due to dysphagia, decubitus ulcers due to immobility.

Breakout Point

- Presents with visual hallucinations, delirium, Parkinsonism, REM sleep disorder
- Relative preservation of memory
- Intracytoplasmic inclusions in neurons

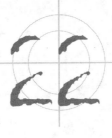

case

ID/CC A **60-year-old woman** says that her family has noted a 1-year history of **marked personality change** and **speech difficulty.**

HPI Her family reports that she is no longer interested in her hobbies of golf and reading. She now becomes angry for no apparent reason. She also hoards shoes.

PE VS: normal. PE: impaired cognitive function; CN II–XII intact; motor strength 5/5, DTRs 2+; prominent snout and grasp reflex noted.

Labs Serum B_{12}, folate, and TSH normal. VDRL: negative.

Imaging MR, brain: marked **bilateral frontotemporal atrophy.**

case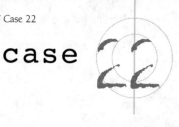

Frontotemporal Dementia (Pick's Disease)

Pathogenesis

Pathologic examination reveals **atrophy** of gray and white matter in the **frontal and temporal lobes.** The characteristic lesions are argentophilic **Pick bodies.**

Management

No specific treatment. The dementia progresses over 3 to 15 years.

Complications

With progression of dementia, complications are primarily **infectious** and include aspiration pneumonia, UTIs, and decubitus ulcers.

Breakout Point

- Atrophy of the frontal and temporal lobes
- Silver staining Pick bodies
- Presents with apathy, emotional lability, disinhibition, hyperorality, lack of insight

case

ID/CC A **60-year-old man** presents with a rapidly progressive **change in mental status** over the past 2 months with an **inability to concentrate** and **memory impairment.**

HPI His relatives have noticed increased somnolence, changes in his personality, **twitching movements of the hands,** and **difficulty walking** (due to ataxia) for several months.

PE VS: normal. PE: no papilledema; normal speech; **ataxic gait** with **choreoathetotic movements** and **myoclonus;** normal DTRs; normal sensation; cranial nerves intact.

Labs CBC/Lytes: normal. TFTs: normal. LFTs: normal. LP: CSF analysis normal. EEG: **diffuse, slow background with superimposed bilateral sharp triphasic synchronous discharge complexes.**

Imaging CT/MR, brain: generalized cortical atrophy.

case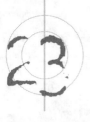

Creutzfeldt–Jakob Disease

Pathogenesis

Creutzfeldt–Jakob disease (CJD) is a **subacute encephalopathy of the spongiform type** that is caused by a slow virus like agent (PRION) with a very long incubation period. CJD gives rise to progressive dementia and associated myoclonus and may be **transmitted** by **corneal transplants, dura mater allografts,** contaminated **cadaveric growth hormone, EEG electrodes,** and **neurosurgical contamination.** Pathologic findings include softening of CNS tissue with vacuolization and secondary amyloidosis but no inflammatory reaction. Unlike Alzheimer's, cerebral atrophy is minimal due to the rapid progression of the disease; 90% die within 1 year. CJD is diagnosed by brain biopsy after other causes of dementia have been ruled out.

Epidemiology

Occurs with greater frequency in the sixth decade of life; shows no gender predominance. Has a higher incidence within families and in certain geographical areas, such as Czechoslovakia, North Africa, and Chile. Between 5 and 15% of cases are autosomal dominant. Closely associated with **kuru from New Guinea,** which is now a rare disease (was transmitted by some tribal traditions of eating human brains).

Management

No specific treatment is available. The disease has a very **poor short-term prognosis.**

Complications

Coma and death.

Breakout Point

> • Subacute spongiform encephalopathy
> • Caused by prion proteins that contain no DNA or RNA
> • Characterized by myoclonus

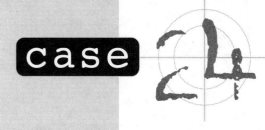

case 24

ID/CC   A **21-year-old man** presents to the emergency room after losing consciousness 30 minutes ago. He has had sustained **rhythmic tonic-clonic contractions of his extremities** since then with eye rolling, tongue biting, and urinary incontinence.

HPI   He has **not regained consciousness** at any point. He has a known **seizure disorder** and has been on **phenytoin.** His girlfriend states that he has been **noncompliant with his medications.** She reports no history of head trauma or injury.

PE   VS: fever (100.8°F); hypertensive (160/70); tachycardic (HR 110); tachypnea (RR 30); SpO$_2$: 90% on 2L O$_2$. PE: unresponsive; generalized tonic-clonic activity with sonorous respirations; eyes deviated upward; **positive lip bite.** Pupils pinpoint and reactive; no papilledema; nonfocal neurological exam.

Labs   CBC: moderate leukocytosis. Lytes: normal, including glucose. **Dilantin level 1.1.** ABGs: metabolic (lactic) acidosis. LP: CSF normal. Blood and urine cultures pending.

Imaging   None.

case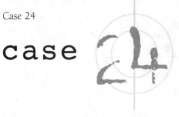

Status Epilepticus

Pathogenesis

Status epilepticus (SE) is a true **neurologic emergency.** Numerous systemic and primary brain changes occur during convulsive SE. Prolonged seizure activity can cause permanent brain damage with pathologic changes after 30 minutes; after 60 minutes, neurons begin to die. The longer SE persists, the more likely those neurons are damaged by excitatory neurotransmitters. Sustained seizure activity also progressively reduces gamma-amino butyric acid (GABA) inhibition.

Epidemiology

About 200,000 new cases of SE occur each year in the United States with 20% mortality. SE occurs at the extremes of age. Subtherapeutic levels of anticonvulsants are a common cause. In children, prolonged fever also commonly causes SE. In adults, SE is often precipitated by strokes or withdrawal of anticonvulsants.

Management

ABCs; thiamine and then glucose; correct electrolytes and give IV saline. **Stop seizure activity:** after about 5 minutes of seizure activity, lorazepam IV. every 2 minutes (max of 8 mg in adults and 4 mg in children) or diazepam. Phenytoin (or fosphenytoin): give even if seizures cease with benzodiazepine administration; if still seizing, then phenobarbital or valproate; if still seizing, then go to pharmacologic coma with EEG pattern of **"burst suppression"** using anesthetics (propofol, midazolam, or pentobarbital).

Complications

Hypotension, arrhythmias, respiratory depression, aspiration, rhabdomyolysis, and death.

Breakout Point

- "Seizures beget seizures."
- Neurologic emergency: maximize with benzodiazepine (lorazepam) initially, then phenytoin or other anticonvulsants, until seizing stops.

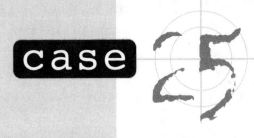

ID/CC   A **16-year-old boy** presents with sudden **loss of consciousness** and muscle hypertonia followed by **rhythmic movements of the limbs** with upward rolling of the eyes, tongue biting, and urinary incontinence; he is now in a state of confusion and lethargy.

HPI   He is otherwise healthy and is a good student. He has two cousins who suffer from a seizure disorder. He does not take any illicit drugs or medications.

PE   VS: normal. PE: lethargic; complains of headache but is awake and oriented; no cyanosis; lesion on anterior third of tongue attributed to bite during seizure; nonfocal neurologic examination.

Labs   CBC/LFTs: normal. Sao_2 99%. Lytes: metabolic acidosis. Elevated serum lactate and CK. UA: toxicology screen negative. **Prolactin elevated** (it does not rise after a psychogenic tonic-clonic "seizure"). ECG: normal sinus rhythm.

Imaging   CT, head: no apparent intracranial pathology.

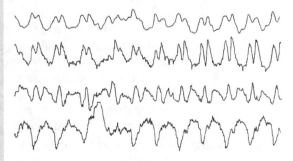

Figure 25-1. EEG: diffuse slowing with generalized spike-and-wave pattern. LP: CSF normal.

case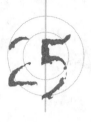

Seizure, Grand Mal

Pathogenesis

Grand mal seizures are also called generalized tonic-clonic seizures. A tonic-clonic seizure can begin as a partial complex seizure, in which case it is termed partial complex seizure secondarily generalized.

Epidemiology

Half of patients who suffer a new-onset tonic-clonic seizure will have a recurrence. Epilepsy may remit spontaneously in up to one-third of cases and may be controlled with medications.

Management

Start with a low dose of **valproic acid** (side effects include severe, fatal hepatotoxicity, pancreatitis, thrombocytopenia, hair loss, GI upset, ataxia, sedation, and tremors) and increase dosage slowly; the vast majority of cases can be controlled with a single drug; if not effective despite therapeutic blood levels, second options include older medications such as **phenytoin** (side effects include numerous drug interactions, gingival hyperplasia, facial coarsening, ataxia, hirsutism, rash, lymphadenopathy, megaloblastic anemia, and osteomalacia) or **carbamazepine** (side effects include GI upset, thrombocytopenia, aplastic anemia, hepatotoxicity, ataxia, vertigo, and diplopia). **Lamotrigine, topiramate,** and **zonisamide** are newer broad-spectrum drugs that may be well tolerated. **Phenobarbital** is classically used but has become less popular recently because of cognitive side effects. When the patient has been seizure-free on medications for 2 years, tapering may be attempted though recurrence is likely.

Complications

Chronicity, difficulty controlling seizure activity, **status epilepticus** (single seizure lasting >30 minutes or a series of seizures with no return to consciousness lasting >30 minutes), and **motor vehicle accidents.**

Breakout Point

- Stereotypic rhythmic movements
- Urinary incontinence
- Prolonged post-ictal confusion
- May occur with no aura or warning

case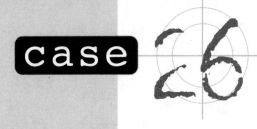

ID/CC A **16-year-old boy** is brought to the physician by his mother, who reports two recent episodes during which she observed her son to be "out of it."

HPI In his first episode, he complained of an unpleasant smell (AURA), suddenly stopped talking, and "**stared straight ahead**"; his mouth was twitching. Each episode was over in approximately 2 minutes, after which the patient was **confused and sleepy** (POSTIC-TAL CONFUSION). After taking a nap, he returned to normal. When he was an infant, he had **herpes encephalitis.** He has required remedial reading and math classes since the third grade. There is no family history of seizures, and the patient denies any alcohol or drug use.

PE VS: normal. PE: no focal neurologic deficits.

Labs CBC: normal. PFTs: SaO_2 99%. Lytes: normal. Toxicology screen negative. EEG: normal background with **focal spike discharges over left temporal lobe**; no frank seizure activity.

Imaging MR, brain: **left mesial temporal sclerosis**; hippocampal calcification.

case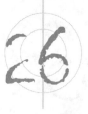

Complex Partial Seizures

Pathogenesis

Complex partial seizures are also referred to as **temporal lobe** or **psychomotor epilepsy.** Unlike simple partial seizures, they always involve loss of consciousness and frequently **follow auditory or olfactory auras.** Medial temporal sclerosis is scar tissue that, in this case, resulted from the patient's childhood encephalitis; **scar tissue serves as a focus for seizure activity.** The cause of most seizure disorders is idiopathic, but birth injuries, head trauma, childhood febrile convulsions, and CNS malignancies can cause seizures. Seizures may occur unpredictably without any precipitating cause. However, external factors that may lower the seizure threshold include lack of sleep, missed meals, stress, alcohol or other drugs, fever, and specific stimuli such as flickering lights.

Epidemiology

Epilepsy shows a **male predominance** and is most common in the first decade of life and then after the age of 60.

Management

Phenytoin and **carbamazepine** are both effective in treating complex partial seizures; the choice of drug is based on its side-effect profile. The primary side effects of phenytoin are gingival hyperplasia, ataxia, lymphadenopathy, various drug interactions, hirsutism, facial coarsening, rash, and osteomalacia; those of carbamazepine are leukopenia, nausea, vomiting, and hepatotoxicity.

Complications

Secondary generalization of seizure that began as a complex partial seizure; serious injury during seizure episode; and **status epilepticus.**

Breakout Point

- Complex partial seizure: aura followed by impaired consciousness
- Cerebral scar tissue may be focus of seizure activity
- Can still make basic verbal responses or follow simple motor commands

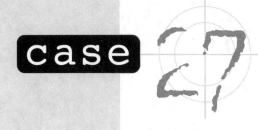

case 27

ID/CC A **4-year-old girl** has been having **episodes of persistent staring** during which she does not answer questions and **looks distracted.**

HPI During the episodes, the child rolls her eyes upward, rhythmically nods her head, and drops objects from her hand. One of the child's cousins has had similar episodes.

PE VS: normal. PE: neurologic exam normal; with hyperventilation and under strobe light, she was shown to have fine, twitching movements of the eyelids, pupillary dilatation (MYDRIASIS), tachycardia, piloerection, and changes in postural tone, including nodding of her head.

Labs CBC: normal. SaO_2 98%. Lytes/LFTs/UA: normal. Calcium normal.

Imaging MR, brain: no organic pathology.

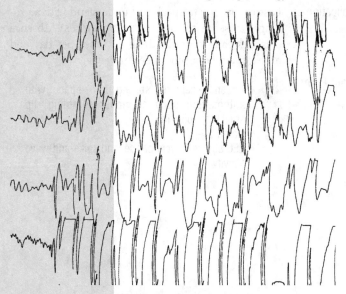

Figure 27-1. EEG: during seizure, **bursts of 3-cycle-per-second spike-and-wave activity** occur; in the interictal period, EEG is normal.

case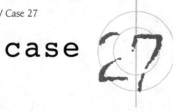

Absence Seizure

Pathogenesis

Also called **petit mal** seizures, absence seizures are inherited as an **autosomal-recessive** trait and are characterized by an idiopathic, temporary (usually <10 seconds) **loss of awareness** that is **not preceded by an aura** and is followed by a characteristic abrupt regaining of consciousness. Hyperventilation, lack of sleep, and blinking strobe lights may precipitate the attacks.

Epidemiology

Higher incidence in children aged 3 to 13 years; more common among girls. Petit mal seizures never begin after age 20.

Management

Most patients show a **benign course,** with symptoms disappearing by puberty. **Ethosuximide** and **valproic acid** are useful drugs; a ketogenic or medium-chain triglyceride diet will also help.

Complications

Loss of capacity to speak and understand with a prolonged absence seizure (PETIT MAL STATUS). Absence episodes can occur hundreds of times per day and may explain poor school performance.

Breakout Point

- Absence seizure: staring into space with automatism such as finger fumbling, lip smacking, blinking
- No aura
- EEG shows 3 cycle-per-second spike-and-wave activity

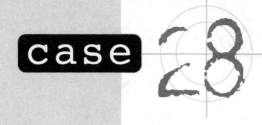

ID/CC A **10-month-old child** is rushed to the emergency room because of sudden loss of consciousness and rigidity of muscles followed by **jerky movements of all limbs, upward rolling of the eyes, and urination.**

HPI The patient was being treated for **severe otitis media** and had a 40.2°C temperature when the seizure began.

PE VS: **fever** (38.1°C). PE: neck supple; pupils equal, round, and reactive to light; no focal neurologic signs; severe otitis media in right ear.

Labs CBC: leukocytosis with left shift. Sao$_2$ 98%. Lytes/UA: normal. LP: CSF normal. EEG: posterior asymmetric slowing of background.

Imaging CT, head: normal.

case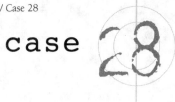

Febrile Seizure

Pathogenesis

Febrile seizures are those that occur in children **younger than 5 years** and **older than 6 months of age,** have **no organic cause,** and are **precipitated by a high fever. Recurrence** occurs more often in children with: seizures at a lower level of fever, a young age of onset, a family history, and marked slowing on EEG.

Epidemiology

There is usually a family history of the disease, and recurrence occurs in 30% of patients.

Management

Temperature control with acetaminophen and cold baths. **Diazepam** may be used in the acute setting to control seizures. Treat a precipitating bacterial infection with appropriate antibiotics.

Complications

Mental deficiency, **developmental disturbances** (especially in patients with previous neurologic disturbance and with focal seizures), status epilepticus, and epilepsy development (rare).

Breakout Point

> Strongly consider LP to rule out bacterial meningitis in children, especially if younger than 12 months (who may have subtle or absent clinical symptoms and signs).

case 29

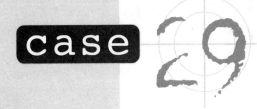

ID/CC	A **66-year-old man** with **lung cancer** is discovered "**shaking**" in bed and unable to speak.
HPI	He was diagnosed with lung cancer 6 months ago and has been treated with chemotherapy (which may transiently weaken the blood-brain barrier [BBB]). He has complained of severe early-morning **headaches** associated with **nausea and projectile vomiting**, which improve as the day progresses, coupled with **blurred vision** (due to papilledema). Now he is **confused,** but his right arm and leg are no longer shaking (POSTICTAL STATE).
PE	VS: normal. PE: drowsy but able to follow commands; **4/5 strength in right** arm and leg with 5/5 strength on left; **bilateral papilledema.**
Labs	CBC: anemia. Lytes: normal. Troponin I normal.
Imaging	CT, head: **ring-enhancing lesion** in the **left parietal region**.

Figure 29-1. CT, head (with contrast): **ring-enhancing lesion** (1) in the **left parietal region** with surrounding mild edema.

case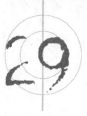

Seizure, Metastatic Disease

Pathogenesis

The metastatic lesion serves as the seizure focus. Symptoms are due to edema surrounding the mass and destruction of brain tissue by the metastases.

Epidemiology

Fifteen percent of patients with diagnosed cancer develop cerebral metastases (40% are single lesions). **Malignancies that commonly metastasize to the brain** are **lung, breast, melanoma, renal cell,** and **colon.**

Management

Begin **lifelong antiepileptic treatment** (e.g., phenytoin). Obtain an MR of the brain to determine the possible presence of one or more metastatic lesions. In the presence of a **single brain lesion** and if the patient is in relatively good health, **resection** will improve life span. If the patient is in poor health or has **multiple metastatic lesions** of the brain, then **radiation** (breast and small cell lung cancer metastases respond well; melanoma and kidney adenocarcinoma metastases are resistant to radiotherapy) and **steroids** (IV dexamethasone) can be used to reduce the edema surrounding the lesion.

Complications

Recurrent seizures (due to scarring or to persistence or further growth of tumor), severe headaches, altered mental status, and increasing neurologic deficits.

Breakout Point

- Ring-enhancing lesion from metastasis
- Many chemotherapeutic agents do not cross the BBB, allowing tumor growth in the brain

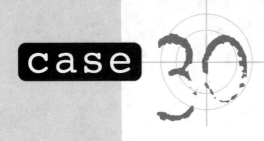

case

ID/CC A **70-year-old woman** presents with a **severe, inter-mittent right temporal headache** and **fever** of 2 months' duration and **blurred vision in the right eye** for 2 days.

HPI The headache is neither relieved nor aggravated by changes in position or activity level. The patient also complains of **pain in the jaw when chewing** (CLAU-DICATION), weight loss, and discomfort on combing the right scalp but denies any associated nausea, vomiting, photophobia, or phonophobia. She has achieved some relief with acetaminophen.

PE VS: mild fever; otherwise normal. PE: visual acuity normal; funduscopy reveals a swollen right disk; pal-pation reveals a right **temporal artery** that is **tender, pulseless, nodular,** and tortuous; locally tender scalp.

Labs CBC: mild normocytic, normochromic **anemia;** mild leukocytosis and thrombocytosis. **Markedly elevated ESR** (>80 mm/h) and C-reactive protein (>2.4); SPEP reveals mild polyclonal hypergammaglobuline-mia; RF, ANA, and dsDNA negative (rules out connec-tive tissue disorders); **temporal artery biopsy reveals mononuclear cell infiltrates in the media,** particu-larly in the internal elastic lamina, as well as intimal thickening and granulomas containing multinucleated giant cells, histiocytes, and lymphocytes.

Imaging None.

case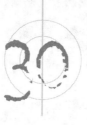

Temporal Arteritis (Giant Cell Arteritis)

Pathogenesis

The etiology of temporal arteritis is unknown. The histopathologic lesion is **giant-cell granuloma** within the vessel wall, leading to stenosis of the lumen. Involvement of an affected artery is patchy. Vascular inflammation is found most often in the superficial temporal arteries as well as in the vertebral, ophthalmic, and posterior ciliary arteries.

Epidemiology

Median age of onset is 75. About five times more prevalent in females.

Management

High-dose corticosteroids urgently to prevent blindness; continue until symptoms resolve and ESR normalizes, and then taper slowly. Most patients require a minimum of 1 to 2 years of therapy; some will require chronic steroid administration. Early temporal artery biopsy yields a definitive diagnosis.

Complications

Loss of vision and opportunistic infections (due to long-term prednisone treatment). Highly associated with aneurysm development, especially in thoracic aorta. Death may occur from strokes, ruptured aorta secondary to aortitis, and MI from coronary arteritis.

Breakout Point

- Should be suspected in any patient >50 years old with new headache
- Presents with headache, jaw claudication, ESR >100, polymyalgia rheumatica
- Immediately start prednisone to prevent blindness

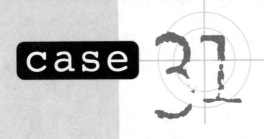

case 27

ID/CC A **21-year-old woman** presents with a history of **intermittent, severe headaches** of 3 years' duration.

HPI She gets headaches approximately six times per year. The headaches begin with light flashes in the right visual field (SCINTILLATION) that last for 15 to 20 minutes; approximately 10 minutes later, a **unilateral** left **temporal throbbing pain** begins. The pain increases in severity and then lasts for 10 to 12 hours. Occasionally the headaches are **associated with nausea and vomiting.** In addition, she cannot bear light, movement, or noise during the episodes. She has a **family history of migraine.**

PE VS: stable. PE: funduscopy reveals sharp disks bilaterally; visual acuity 20/20 bilaterally; remainder of neurologic exam normal.

Labs CBC/Lytes: normal. ESR: normal (to evaluate for temporal arteritis).

Imaging None.

HEADACHE

case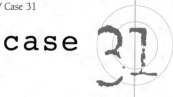

Classic Migraine (Migraine with Aura)

Pathogenesis

Individuals have noted various **precipitants** to migraines, including red wine, exercise, menstruation, estrogen, caffeine, lack of sleep, and skipping of meals. Migraine can occur with **aura** (a transient neurologic dysfunction, usually visual in nature, which occurs minutes before headache onset).

Epidemiology

Most commonly, the initial attack is during **teenage years.** Migraine without aura (common migraine) is more common than migraine with aura (classic migraine). More **common in females** after puberty.

Management

Prophylaxis with **beta-blockers, verapamil,** or **valproic acid. Abortive treatment** consists of **NSAIDs, sumatriptan,** and **dihydroergotamine nasal spray.**

Breakout Point

- Throbbing lateralized headache, nausea, vomiting, photophobia, phonophobia
- Aura of flashes or zigzags of light (scotoma) may occur

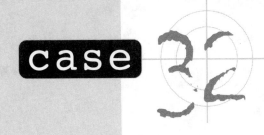

case

ID/CC	A **26-year-old man** complains of having "**terrible headaches**" for the past 5 years.
HPI	The headaches usually occur at night and generally start with a **burning in the right eye** that, within minutes, involves the right orbit and right temple. The pain feels like a "hot poker" behind the right eye; the right eye then starts **tearing** and the **right nostril begins to run.** The pain lasts for 45 minutes. The patient generally has **three to four attacks within a 24-hour period every 6 months.** He states that the **symptoms usually occur after** consumption of **alcohol.**
PE	VS: normal. PE: leonine facial appearance; neurologic exam normal; **lacrimation** from right eye; during an acute episode, ptosis, miosis, anhidrosis, and enophthalmos of the right eye are present (HORNER'S SYNDROME).
Labs	CBC: normal. ESR: normal.
Imaging	MR/CT, brain: no intracranial lesion or hemorrhage; no significant abnormality.

case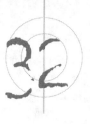

Cluster Headache

Pathogenesis

The pathology of cluster headache is thought to be vascular in nature. The neurotransmitter **substance P** may mediate the pain.

Epidemiology

Cluster headaches usually occur in **patients in their 20s** and are much more common in **males**; patients commonly have a **smoking history.** Many patients report that attacks **occur at the same time of year** (e.g., January and July).

Management

Prophylactic treatment consists of **verapamil** or **methysergide** for 1 to 2 months (methysergide increases risk of retroperitoneal fibrosis and can be only given for limited periods). **Prednisone, ergotamine,** and **lithium** are also used for prophylactic treatment. **Abortive therapy** consists of **100% high-flow oxygen** at 8 to 10 L/min, **intranasal lidocaine,** or **sumatriptan.**

Complications

Recurrence and persistence into late life.

Breakout Point

- Occurs in middle-aged men
- Occurs at night, lasts for <2 hours
- Severe lateralized periorbital headache with ipsilateral nasal congestion, lacrimation, conjunctival hyperemia, facial diaphoresis, and Horner syndrome
- Occurs in "clusters"

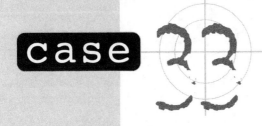

ID/CC   A **62-year-old housewife** complains of **recurrent episodes of headaches** that she has experienced since the age of 40.

HPI   Initially, her headaches presented as a moderate **squeezing pain** in the **bilateral frontal area.** The headaches occurred twice monthly and were relieved with two acetaminophen tablets and a nap. For the past 2 years, the headaches have occurred three to four times a week, with accompanying nausea approximately one to two times a week. Minimal relief is obtained with ibuprofen. She denies associated phonophobia, photophobia, or focal motor deficits.

PE   VS: normal. PE: funduscopic exam reveals sharp disks bilaterally; visual acuity 20/20 bilaterally; neurologic exam normal.

Labs   ESR: normal.

Imaging   CT, head: no intracranial lesions or hemorrhage.

HEADACHE

case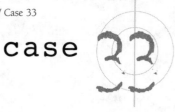

Tension Headache

Pathogenesis

Chronic tension headache is characterized by pain that is **bilateral** in location and present for **more than 15 days per month** for at least the last **6 months;** it may or may not be accompanied by nausea, and there is no vomiting or photophobia. Pain is rarely throbbing in nature and is not aggravated by routine physical activity. Tension headache typically occurs at the end of the day; migraines can occur at any time. Overuse of OTC medications or depression may play a role.

Management

Add **amitriptyline** or gabapentin to **NSAIDs** or **acetaminophen.** To determine efficacy, 4 to 6 weeks of treatment is necessary.

Complications

Recurrent headaches.

Breakout Point

- Most common type of headache
- "Vise-like" daily headaches, exacerbated by stress, fatigue, noise

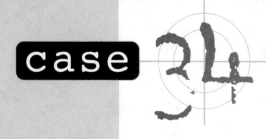

case 24

ID/CC	An **18-year-old woman** complains of **headache, vomiting,** and **blurred vision** for the past 2 to 3 weeks.
HPI	She experiences the headache as a "pressure-like" feeling in the parietal region bilaterally. She also experienced intermittent brief loss of vision while bending. She denies any associated photophobia or phonophobia.
PE	VS: normal. PE: **obese; bilateral papilledema;** neck supple; neurologic exam otherwise normal.
Labs	CBC: normal. LP: **opening pressure elevated** (34 cm H_2O); no white cells; normal protein and glucose.
Imaging	CT, head: no mass, hemorrhage, or midline shift; normal ventricle size (may even be small). MR, venography: narrowing of the transverse dural venous sinus (possibly a result of increased ICP); however, no transverse and sagittal sinus thrombosis.

HEADACHE

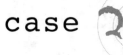 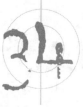

Pseudotumor Cerebri

Pathogenesis
Pseudotumor cerebri, also known as idiopathic (or benign) intracranial hypertension, is an idiopathic condition; **overproduction of CSF** and **impairment of CSF absorption** by the arachnoid villi may be involved. Pseudotumor can follow corticosteroid withdrawal or excesses of vitamin A or tetracycline. Obesity may increase intra-abdominal pressure and subsequently result in impeded venous return.

Epidemiology
Incidence is higher in **obese women** between the **childbearing ages** of 15 and 44.

Management
Withdrawal of precipitating agent. Weight loss may reduce recurrence. Treatment with **acetazolamide** causes decreased CSF production and lowers ICP; if not tolerated, **furosemide** may be used. Severe (e.g., visual loss) or refractory cases may require a short course of high-dose corticosteroids (e.g., **prednisone**). **Serial LPs** have a role if no medications can be tolerated. If **visual loss** continues despite medical therapy, then consider optic nerve sheath fenestration or **CSF shunting.**

Complications
Optic atrophy causing **permanent visual loss**; electrolyte abnormalities due to diuretic therapy.

Breakout Point
- Presents as headache, papilledema, diplopia (CN VI dysfunction) in a young obese female
- May evolve into visual loss if untreated

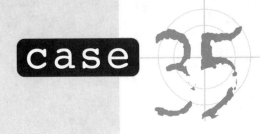

case 35

ID/CC A **60-year-old man** complains of the development of a **hand tremor** coupled with **generalized muscle rigidity**.

HPI His wife has noted generalized slowing of movement (BRADYKINESIA) and **lack of facial expression** (MASK-LIKE FACIES) together with drooling. He has also noticed that his handwriting has been getting smaller (MICROGRAPHIA). The involuntary tremor decreases during voluntary motion.

PE VS: normal. PE: severe seborrhea of scalp (indicative of autonomic dysfunction); sustained blinking follows tapping on nasal bridge (MYERSON'S SIGN); stooped posture; **postural instability; gait short- and slow-stepped** at first, followed by quick forward steps to prevent fall (FESTINANT GAIT), with no arm swing; intermittent muscle spasms with passive movement of joints (COGWHEEL RIGIDITY); asymmetric, pill-rolling **resting tremor** of right hand; DTRs normal; flexor plantar responses.

Labs ESR: normal. Lytes/LFTs: normal. TSH: normal.

Imaging CXR/KUB: within normal limits.

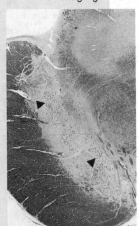

Figure 35-1. Substantia nigra, showing normal population of large pigmented cells.

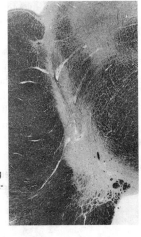

Figure 35-2. Severe depletion of pigmented cells), specifically the substantia nigra, which shows loss of pigmentation on postmortem analysis.

case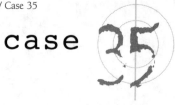

Parkinson's Disease

Pathogenesis

Parkinson's disease is characterized by **loss of dopaminergic neurons in the basal ganglia.** It is usually idiopathic but also may occur after influenza infections, following CO or manganese poisoning, after exposure to the drug **MPTP** (an impurity found in poorly synthesized heroin), with antipsychotic drugs, with basal ganglia tumors, following trauma, and after episodes of encephalitis (POSTEN-CEPHALITIC PARKINSONISM).

Epidemiology

A common disorder (1 per 1,000 population) that usually has an onset between 45 and 65 years of age (1 per 100 in people older than 65).

Management

Levodopa crosses the blood-brain barrier (BBB) and is converted to dopamine in the CNS (side effects include dyskinesia, arrhythmias, nausea, vomiting, hypotension, and psychosis). It is usually administered with **carbidopa** (a dopamine decarboxylase inhibitor that does not cross the BBB) to reduce the required dose of L-dopa and limit side effects. **Anticholinergics** are given for their beneficial effect on rigidity and tremors (side effects include dry mouth, blurring of vision, urinary retention, and exacerbation of glaucoma). **Amantadine** is used for mild disease, although its mechanism of action is not well understood (side effects include depression, anxiety, constipation, arrhythmias, and postural hypotension). **Bromocriptine** is a dopamine agonist associated with a lesser incidence of dyskinesia (side effects include digital vasospasm, nasal congestion, constipation, and worsening of peptic ulcer disease). **Selegiline** is an MAO-B inhibitor that prevents the breakdown of dopamine in the brain. **Surgery** includes implantation of adrenal medulla in the caudate nucleus, thalamotomy, or pallidotomy with variable results. **Deep brain stimulation** is emerging as an alternative to surgical treatment.

Complications

Progressive disability and death.

Breakout Point

- Resting tremor (asymmetric)
- Rigidity (lead pipe or cogwheel)
- Bradykinesia (e.g. micrographia, decreased facial expression, decreased blink rate, and soft speech)

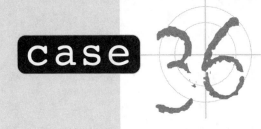
ID/CC   A **38-year-old woman** presents with a 1-year history of progressively worsening **abrupt, involuntary jerking movements** of the limbs (CHOREA), absentmindedness, and slurred speech.

HPI   Her family first noted her inability to button clothes. Movements began with facial twitches and now are coarse, **purposeless, dance-like movements of the extremities** that disappear during sleep. Family members also complain that the patient is depressed, irritable, impulsive, and emotionally labile. For the past 6 months, she has displayed memory impairment. Her **mother died of "dementia"** at the age of 55, and her **brother was placed in a nursing home** at the age of 48.

PE   VS: normal. PE: blunted affect; unable to follow complex (three-step) commands; **lack of verbal and perceptual skills; deficits in attention,** organization, and sequencing abilities (due to frontal system dysfunction); short-term memory defective; diminished muscle tone.

Labs   **Trinucleotide repeat** in Huntington gene on chromosome 4p.

Imaging   CT, head: bilateral cerebral atrophy; rounding (due to caudate atrophy) and enlargement of the anterior horns of the lateral ventricles.

MOVEMENT

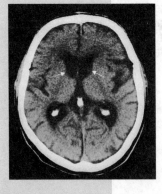

Figure 36-1. CT, head: bilateral cerebral atrophy; rounding (due to caudate atrophy) and enlargement of the anterior horns of the lateral ventricles.

case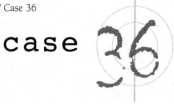

Huntington's Disease

Pathogenesis

An **autosomal-dominant** condition with **high penetrance** characterized by widespread loss of neurons in the neostriatum, Huntington's disease is an **incurable,** chronic, progressive neurodegenerative disorder. The function of the Huntington gene and its product is unknown. Successive generations exhibit **lengthening of the trinucleotide (CAG) repeat** (GENETIC ANTICIPATION) and thus experience onset at progressively **younger ages.**

Epidemiology

Symptoms usually begin between 35 and 45 years. The mean age of death is in the mid-50s.

Management

No treatment is available for the underlying neurologic disease. **Haloperidol,** perphenazine, or drugs that **block dopamine receptors** or **deplete brain monoamines** reduce choreiform movements. Tricyclic antidepressants or SSRIs for depression. Broach with the patient the topic of disclosing the diagnosis to immediate relatives so they may undergo genetic testing.

Complications

Patients may develop dysphagia and become progressively rigid and bedridden. Death is typically due to infections such as pneumonia or UTI.

Breakout Point

- Autosomal dominant inheritance
- Trinucleotide repeat disorder
- Movement (chorea progressing to dystonia, parkinsonian features and eventually akinesia)
- Cognition (dementia)
- Behavior (e.g. affective illness and suicide)

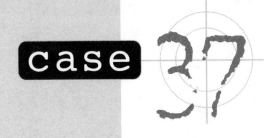
ID/CC   A **9-year-old boy** was brought to the clinic by his parents due to **unusual movements** and **vocalizations**.

HPI   He has a history of **obsessive–compulsive personality disorder.** Two years ago, he started having **stereotyped involuntary** facial grimacing, quick jerky head turns, and shoulder shrugs, which worsen when he is under stress and disappear during sleep. He can voluntarily suppress the movements, but doing so results in an overwhelming degree of anxiety, which can only be relieved by movement. One year ago, he started having **involuntary vocalizations,** such as clearing his throat, grunting, and snorting.

PE   He appears very nervous. He occasionally shrugs his shoulder, jerks his head to the side, grimaces his face, repeatedly clears his throat (VOCAL AND MOTOR TICS). The rest of his neurologic examination is unremarkable.

Labs   CBC, BMP, LFTs, and TFTs are all normal.

Imaging   MRI, brain: normal.

MOVEMENT

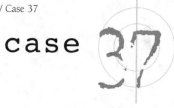

case 37

Gilles de la Tourette's Syndrome

Pathogenesis

Gilles de la Tourette's syndrome is characterized by chronic **multiple motor and vocal tics. Tics** are rapid, repetitive stereotyped movements that may be simple, brief jerks, which typically begin between the ages of 2 and 21 years. The onset of motor tics often precedes vocal tics, and they typically involve the head first and extend caudally. Simple tics may progress to complex tics including **echopraxia** (imitation of others' movements), **coprolalia** (vulgar or obscene speech), **echolalia** (repeating speech of others), and **palilalia** (repetition of words and phrases). **Comorbid conditions** such as **obsessive–compulsive disorder (OCD) and attention deficit disorder** are common. Increased D_2 receptor activity in the caudate nucleus may play a role in generating this disorder.

Epidemiology

Boys are far more commonly affected than girls. The prevalence of the disorder is 5 in 10,000 persons. The disorder is often sporadic, although there are rare familial cases where the inheritance is autosomal dominant.

Management

Symptomatic treatment using **clonidine** which decreases the noradrenergic output from neurons in the locus ceruleus and **Haloperidol,** a dopamine blocking agent.

Complications

Depression and suicide related to social embarrassment.

Breakout Point

- Motor and vocal tics
- Often have comorbid OCD

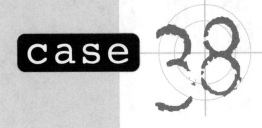

case 28

ID/CC	A **65-year-old right-handed woman** with a history of **hypertension** presents with sudden, uncontrollable movements of the right arm and leg.
HPI	When working in her garden, she suddenly became unable to plant flowers, as she could not control the movements of her right arm. She was well before this episode.
PE	VS: normal. PE: rapid, irregular, and **violent flinging movements of the right arm,** worse proximally. Right leg shows similar but much milder movements.
Labs	CBC, BMP, LFTs, PT, and PTT are all normal.
Imaging	MRI, brain: a small acute infarct in the region of the **left subthalamic nucleus.**

MOVEMENT

case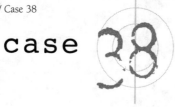

Hemiballismus

Pathogenesis

Hemiballism comes from the Greek word for throwing and often results from a lesion in the contralateral **subthalamic nucleus** or its connections. In older adults, strokes of the basal ganglia may cause focal destructive lesions of the subthalamic nucleus, leading to reduced inhibition of the thalamus and involuntary movements of the **contralateral** limbs.

Epidemiology

Hemiballism is a relatively rare hyperkinetic disorder. Stroke is the most common cause, responsible for more than half of cases.

Management

Hemiballism following stroke usually improves over months and responds to treatment with **dopamine blocking agents** such as haloperidol or dopamine depleters. Medically refractory cases can be treated using **stereotactic thalamotomy.**

Complications

Untreated violent hemiballismus is functionally disabling to patients. It also can cause exhaustion and injury due to falls.

Breakout Point

- Results from lesion in the contralateral sub-thalamic nucleus

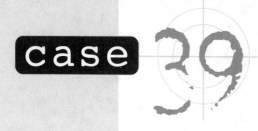

case 39

ID/CC A **28-year-old woman** complains of **occasional double vision** and **"droopy" eyelids.**

HPI For the past 3 months, she has noted intermittent diplopia that arises when she exerts herself. Her husband adds that her **eyelids become droopy at night but are normal in the morning.**

PE VS: normal. PE: **bilateral ptosis** that **worsens with repeated blinking;** extraocular muscles intact, with diplopia on extremes of lateral gaze; motor strength 5/5 bilaterally on initial and 4/5 on prolonged testing; DTRs normal; sensory exam normal.

Labs **Elevated acetylcholine receptor antibody** titer; anti-MuSK (muscle-specific kinase) antibody titer. EMG: decrease in muscle action potential with repeated firing. **Tensilon** test (IV injection of acetylcholinesterase inhibitor) leads to resolution of ptosis and diplopia on lateral gaze.

Imaging CT, chest: lobular **thymic mass** in the anterior mediastinum.

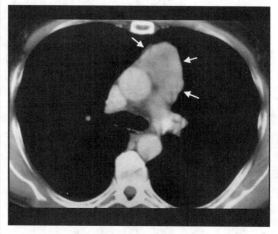

Figure 39-1. CT, chest: lobular **thymic mass** in the anterior mediastinum.

case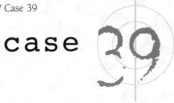

Myasthenia Gravis

Pathogenesis

Myasthenia gravis is an **autoimmune process** that causes **skeletal muscle weakness** and **fatigability on exertion.** Antibodies are produced to the acetylcholine receptor (AchR), resulting in the destruction of receptors and disruption of the neuromuscular junction (NMJ). It can be distinguished clinically from Eaton–Lambert syndrome by **worsening rather than improving symptoms with repetitive motion.**

Epidemiology

Myasthenia gravis has a prevalence of approximately 1 in 7,000, with a peak incidence in younger women and older men.

Management

Pyridostigmine, a cholinesterase inhibitor, is used for symptomatic relief of weakness. Treat acute exacerbations with **plasmapheresis** and IV **immunoglobulin.** Long-term **immunosuppression** with corticosteroids and azathioprine. **Thymectomy** may help up to 85% of patients.

Complications

Myasthenic crisis is an acute exacerbation involving respiratory muscles that may require mechanical ventilation; it is often secondary to underlying infection.

Breakout Point

- Anti-AChR antibodies destroy postsynaptic AChR at the NMJ; inhibition of AChE increases ACh concentration at the NMJ
- Edrophonium (short-acting AChE inhibitor) (Tensilon) test to diagnose MG
- May have coexisting thymoma
- Ptosis and muscle weakness worse at the end of the day or with use

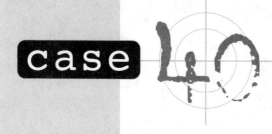

case 40

ID/CC A **64-year-old man** presents with difficulty standing up and walking. The **weakness appears to improve with continued activity.** It has slowly progressed over many weeks.

HPI He also complains of **cough and shortness of breath** for more than 2 years. The cough has been productive and, more recently, with **blood-tinged sputum.** He has had a 25 lb **weight loss** over 6 months. He also has a **history of smoking** for over 40 years.

PE VS: normal. Appears slightly **cachectic.** DTRs are hypoactive. Sensory exam is normal. Motor exam reveals lower extremity weakness (proximal > distal) that improves to normal with repetition. **A monophonic wheeze** is heard over the right chest around the fifth intercostal space. **Clubbing** of digits.

Labs Normal acetylcholine receptor antibody titer. **Elevated voltage-gated calcium channel antibody** titer. EMG: increase in muscle action potential with repeated firing. **Tensilon** test (IV injection of acetylcholinesterase inhibitor) does not dramatically improve strength.

Imaging CXR: A speculated cavitary mass is seen in the right upper lobe.

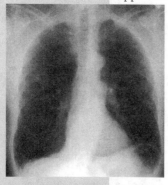

Figure 40-1. CXR: a speculated cavitary mass is seen in the right upper lobe.

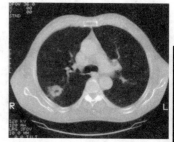

Figure 40-2. CT Chest, noncontrast: cavitary nodule is seen in the right upper lobe.

case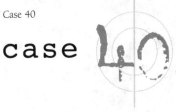

Lambert Eaton Myasthenic Syndrome—Lung Cancer

Pathogenesis

Lambert Eaton Myasthenic Syndrome (LEMS) is an autoimmune process. **Antibodies against voltage gated calcium channels** (VGCC) at the presynaptic terminal result in impaired acetylcholine (ACh) function. This is in contrast to myasthenia gravis, where ACh receptor antibodies are common. Symptoms of weakness often **precede** potential tumor symptoms. The diagnosis is made by demonstration of a **characteristic incremental response to repetitive nerve stimulation** (which is opposite to the response in myasthenia gravis).

Epidemiology

Sixty percent of **small cell** lung cancer patients may have LEMS. **More common in men** than women (2:1), but incidence is rising in women.

Management

Pyridostigmine may be attempted to relieve weakness; prednisone, plasma exchange, IVIG also may be considered in concert with chemotherapy if appropriate. Treatment of underlying cancer; if no known cancer, search for possible occult malignancy. Surgery mainly an adjuvant.

Complications

Compression syndromes associated with lung carcinoma are as follows. **Pancoast tumor: superior sulcus tumor** invading **brachial plexus (C7, C8, T1), stellate ganglion—Horner's syndrome** (ptosis, miosis, anhidrosis, and apparent enophthalmos), **rib destruction**, and atrophy and pain of hand muscles. **Superior vena cava (SVC) syndrome:** compression of SVC as it passes through the thoracic inlet; plethora, venous distention, and edema in the upper thorax, face, and neck. **Recurrent laryngeal nerve compression: hoarseness of the voice;** more **common on the left** side due to a longer intrathoracic course.

Breakout Point

- Anti-calcium channel antibodies result in impaired presynaptic ACh release
- Paraneoplastic disease associated with lung cancer
- Muscle weakness improves with activity or use

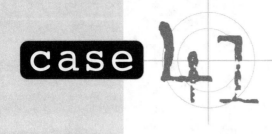

case 47

ID/CC A **77-year-old man** presents with 12 hours of **droopy eyes, double vision, dry mouth,** and **difficulty swallowing.**

HPI He ate **canned beans** for dinner the night before and then started to have nausea, vomiting, and diarrhea, followed by the above symptoms.

PE VS: afebrile. PE: eye exam is notable for **bilateral ptosis** and **dilated pupils** which react sluggishly to light bilaterally. **Facial weakness, dysarthria,** soft speech (HYPOPHONIA), diminished gag reflex, and weak tongue protrusion. Mild weakness of neck flexion and shoulder abduction. Sensation is intact.

Labs CBC/Lytes: normal. Blood and stool samples are sent for culture and toxicology.

Imaging MRI, brain: normal.

case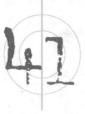

Botulism

Pathogenesis

Botulism is a potentially fatal disease caused by a toxin produced by the anaerobic, spore-forming, Gram-positive bacillus *Clostridium botulinum*. **Food-borne botulism** is transmitted through direct ingestion of the toxin, often in **home-canned** vegetables. **Infant botulism** is produced by ingestion of *C. botulinum* spores, and a history of **honey** ingestion is frequently present. **Wound botulism** is vanishingly rare, and principally affects intravenous drug abusers. Iatrogenic botulism occurs as a side effect of therapeutic injection of botulinum toxin. After an acute gastrointestinal illness, cranial nerves are affected early. Oculobulbar dysfunction is followed by **weakness** that progresses in a **descending** fashion, first involving the arms, then the legs, causing a **flaccid paralysis.** The toxin binds irreversibly to **presynaptic** terminals and **prevents the release of acetylcholine** at the neuromuscular and autonomic nerve junctions. Stool and serum may demonstrate the toxin or the organism. Clinically, botulism is differentiated from myasthenia gravis due to involvement of the pupils. Repetitive nerve stimulation is a neurophysiologic technique that can be helpful to establish a diagnosis of botulism.

Epidemiology

Food-borne botulism constitutes approximately 1,000 annual cases worldwide. There are approximately 30 to 40 cases in the United States per year.

Management

Administer **antitoxin** immediately; although it may prevent the development of further weakness, it cannot reverse existing deficits. Mechanical ventilation and supportive care in an intensive care setting is required, and recovery is often prolonged, requiring several months.

Complications

Respiratory failure, total limb paralysis.

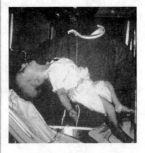

Figure 41-1. A young child with botulism, evident as a marked loss of muscle tone, especially in the region of the head and neck.

Breakout Point

- Toxin inhibits presynaptic ACh release
- Oculobulbar dysfunction followed by descending flaccid paralysis
- The **D's**: **d**ry mouth, **d**iplopia, **d**ilated pupils, **d**ysphonia, **d**ysarthria, **d**ysphagia, **d**roopy eyes, **d**roopy face, **d**escending weakness, **d**iaphragmatic weakness

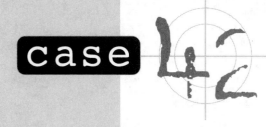

case 42

ID/CC	A **66-year-old man** presents with 6 months of muscle **weakness** in both arms and legs.
HPI	He has had **trouble rising out of a chair** and **lifting his arms** to put away dishes in the cupboards. He has developed a **pruritic rash** over his face, neck, chest, and hands, and has been mildly **short of breath** for the last month.
PE	VS: normal. PE: skin—**erythematous rash** involving his **forehead, malar region, chest, and neck. Papules** are present on the extensor surfaces of his fingers. **Symmetric** moderate **weakness** of the **proximal muscles** of the extremities, particularly the deltoids and iliopsoas bilaterally, but **distal strength is maintained.** Weakness of the **neck flexors.** Reflexes and sensation are normal.
Labs	CBC/Lytes: normal. Serum **CK** highly elevated (2450 IU/L). **ANA** positive. Antibody testing reveals the presence of **anti-Jo-1 antibodies.**
Imaging	None.

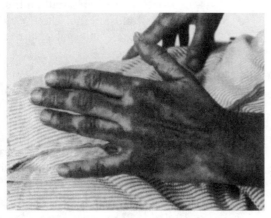

Figure 42-1. Linear extensor erythema and Gottron papules on the knuckles.

NEUROMUSCULAR

case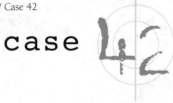

Dermatomyositis

Pathogenesis

Dermatomyositis is an **idiopathic inflammatory myopathy** characterized by **proximal muscle weakness,** skin rash, multiple organ involvement, and an increased risk for malignancy. Serum **creatine kinase** are often **elevated** during the course of the disease, and may precede clinical signs. The characteristic rash is described as **heliotrope** (violet in color), and affects the **forehead, malar regions, chest, neck, and extensor surfaces** of the joints and extremities. **Gottron's papules** are scaly, erythematous lesions found on the extensor surfaces of the digits. Other organs that may be involved include the heart, lungs, and gastrointestinal tract. Patients often demonstrate autoantibodies to nuclear antigens (**ANA**) and **anti-Jo-1** antibodies have been associated with **interstitial lung disease.**

Epidemiology

The estimated incidence of dermatomyositis and polymyositis is 5.5 cases per million.

Management

Corticosteroids are the mainstay of treatment; **Methotrexate** and **azathioprine** can be added if corticosteroids are not effective or if side effects from steroids are intolerable. Screen for an underlying malignancy.

Complications

Side effects from chronic steroid use (steroid-induced myopathy) and pulmonary involvement, which worsen prognosis.

Breakout Point

- Difficulty going up stairs or getting up from chair (proximal muscle weakness)
- Heliotrope rash and Gottron papules are pathognomonic skin manifestations
- Increased risk of malignancy

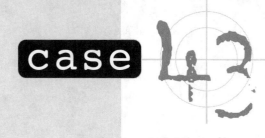

case 42

ID/CC	A **4-year-old boy** presents with 3 months of **clumsy walking** and **frequent falls**.
HPI	He was normal at birth and met his previous motor milestones at the expected ages. His mother noticed a **waddling gait**, which differed from his older sister at that age.
PE	VS: normal. PE: **hypertrophied calves.** A waddling gait due to symmetric weakness of the shoulder and hip girdles with particular weakness in the biceps, quadriceps, and tibialis anterior muscles. When rising from a seated position from the floor, he demonstrates **Gower's sign,** as he cannot stand up without using his arms to support himself. No fasciculations. Reflexes and sensation are normal.
Labs	CBC/Lytes: normal. **CK highly elevated** (12,600 IU/L). Genetic testing shows **absence of dystrophin** gene (75% of cases).
Imaging	None.

case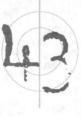

Duchenne Muscular Dystrophy

Pathogenesis

Duchenne muscular dystrophy (DMD) is an **X-linked recessive** disorder, and therefore affects **males** almost exclusively. On muscle biopsy, the muscle-cell membrane protein dystrophin nears complete absence. Children with DMD are normal at birth, develop weakness between ages 2 and 6, are confined to wheelchairs by their early teen years, and usually die of respiratory complications by their early 20s. Weakness is predominantly **proximal** and affects the **lower extremities** more than the upper extremities. Characteristic of DMD is **Gowers' sign,** in which children need to use their arms to rise from the floor to a standing position. **Pseudohypertrophy** of the **calves** is also a classical clinical feature as the muscle is replaced by fibrotic and fatty tissue. DMD is also associated with cardiac dysrhythmias, congestive heart failure, and borderline low intelligence. Becker's muscular dystrophy is a milder form in which the dystrophin protein is abnormal but not absent and patients remain ambulatory through their teens.

Epidemiology

The most frequent childhood-onset myopathy occurring in 1 in 3,500 live male births. The milder form, Becker's muscular dystrophy has an approximate incidence of 1 in 30,000 live male births.

Management

No cure; corticosteroids are the treatment of choice. Physical therapy, bracing, and assistive devices are also required to improve quality of life and prevent contractures.

Complications

Progressive weakness until wheelchair-bound; scoliosis and contractures due to progressive muscle weakness and immobility. Inevitable pulmonary failure requiring mechanical ventilatory support and secretion management.

Breakout Point

- X-linked recessive, affects boys
- Dystrophin deficiency
- Pseudohypertrophy of the calves, proximal muscle weakness (Gowers' sign)

ID/CC A **34-year-old man** presents with **clumsiness of the hands** and multiple "falls."

HPI He is the only child of a **mother who died from a "heart attack"** at the age of 40. He has had increasing difficulty using tools, buttoning shirts, and tying his shoes. He has also begun to trip on the rugs at home. He has **difficulty releasing his grip** when shaking hands.

PE VS: normal. PE: marked **frontal baldness; bilateral ptosis** with hollowing of masseter and temples (HATCHET FACE) and **bilateral facial weakness** (FISH MOUTH); eye exam is notable for cataracts; testicular atrophy; percussion of thenar eminence produces abduction of thumb and firm contraction of thenar eminence (MYOTONIA); bilateral foot drop; weakness and difficulty relaxing distal muscles; sensory exam normal; DTRs reduced.

Labs CBC: normal. Mildly elevated CK; **DNA analysis** reveals 100 copies of a **trinucleotide repeat in the myotonin gene.** EMG: **myotonic discharges.** Muscle biopsy reveals increased number of central nuclei, prominent ring fibers, and areas of disorganized sarcoplasm devoid of normal striations. ECG: **first-degree heart block.**

Imaging None.

case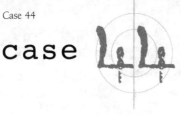

Myotonic Muscular Dystrophy

Pathogenesis

Myotonic dystrophy is inherited as an **autosomal-dominant** disorder. The defect consists of greater than 30 copies of a trinucleotide repeat in the myotonin gene; the function of the myotonin protein is, however, unknown. **Anticipation,** the phenomenon in which successive generations experience more severe disease, is due to expansion in the number of trinucleotide repeats from one generation to the next.

Epidemiology

Incidence is 13.5 in 100,000 live births. The most common muscular dystrophy seen among adults.

Management

Administer **mexiletine** to relieve myotonia. Use orthotic devices to alleviate foot drop. **Cardiac evaluation,** as there is a high incidence of **arrhythmias.**

Complications

Sudden death due to cardiac conduction defects; cataracts; and testicular atrophy.

Breakout Point

- Autosomal dominant inheritance
- Muscle contraction followed by delayed muscle relaxation
- Cannot release handgrip after shaking hands

case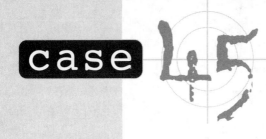

ID/CC	A **55-year-old man** presents with a **generalized seizure.**
HPI	He has never had a seizure before. He has experienced **headaches** that are worse in the morning and admits to occasional **nausea and vomiting.**
PE	VS: **hypertension** (BP 150/90). PE: exhibits confusion; neck supple; **bilateral papilledema; Babinski's sign present on right side;** normal lung and skin exam.
Labs	CBC: normal.
Imaging	CT, head: single, irregular enhancing left temporoparietal mass lesion with necrotic center, mass effect, and moderate surrounding edema.

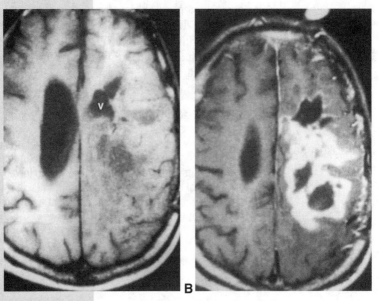

Figure 45-1. MRI, brain: in another patient, a large mass of low-intensity signal compressing the left lateral ventricle.

case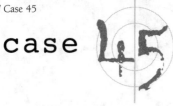

Glioblastoma Multiforme

Pathogenesis

Glioblastoma multiforme (GBM) is a **grade 4 astrocytoma** and is **markedly anaplastic.** Almost 75% of adult brain tumors are **supratentorial,** and the rest are in the posterior fossa. Histopathology reveals abundant necrosis. Metastases are uncommon. Unfortunately, patients with GBM have a very poor prognosis with a median **survival of about 12 months.**

Epidemiology

GBM is the most common glial tumor. The incidence is approximately 2 to 3 new cases per 100,000 people per year. It affects adults mostly, with a peak incidence at 45 to 70 years.

Management

Workup for GBM includes head CT, head MRI, and stereotactic biopsy. Medical treatment includes **corticosteroids** to decrease the edema and anticonvulsants for patients with seizures. Initial treatment of choice is maximal surgical resection without causing major morbidity. Adjuvant radiotherapy and chemotherapy have shown to improve survival.

Complications

Hydrocephalus, seizures, herniation, and functional loss.

Breakout Point

- Most common and most malignant brain tumor
- Presents with signs of increased ICP followed by focal deficits
- Maximal surgical resection, radiation, and chemotherapy

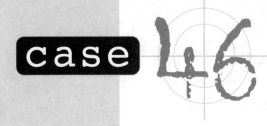

case 46

ID/CC	A **10-year-old boy** presents with a **severe headache** that does not respond to analgesics, along with **projectile vomiting.**
HPI	In the ER, he suffered a **seizure.** The headache was present upon awakening. Directed questioning reveals that he has been behaving oddly for the past month.
PE	VS: normal. PE: appears confused; **ataxic gait; bilateral papilledema;** mild hypotonia of left arm; cardiopulmonary and abdominal exams normal.
Labs	CBC: normal. Sao$_2$ 99%. Lytes: normal. UA: normal. LP/LFTs: normal. TFTs: normal.
Imaging	CT, head: enhancing, irregular **cerebellar mass.**
Pathology	Compact fibrillated cells with microcysts and eosinophilic structures (Rosenthal fibers), consistent with juvenile pilocytic astrocytoma.

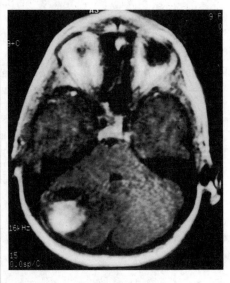

Figure 46-1. MR, brain: partly cystic, partly solid cerebellar astrocytoma.

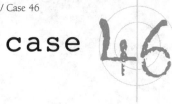

case 46

Astrocytoma

Pathogenesis | Astrocytomas are primary CNS tumors with character-istics of astrocytes. Less aggressive types such as pilo-cytic astrocytoma have a small zone of penetration, whereas low-grade astrocytoma, anaplastic astrocy-tomas have a large area of penetration. Low-grade astrocytomas can transform to high-grade astrocy-tomas over time. High-grade astrocytomas have a very poor prognosis. Risk factors include genetic abnormal-ities such as NF1 and P53 mutations, and prior irradi-ation to the brain.

Epidemiology | Pilocytic astrocytoma generally occurs before age 20. The peak incidence of low-grade astrocytomas occurs in people aged 30 to 40 years.

Management | CT and MRI of the brain are helpful in diagnosis and evaluation. In patients with **high ICP,** avoid LP due to possible downward herniation of the brain. Treatment generally involves **surgical resection,** with possible **adjuvant chemotherapy** and **radio-therapy** for aggressive disease.

Complications | **Hydrocephalus, seizures,** herniation, functional loss, and irradiation damage (neuropsychological dis-turbances, hypothyroidism, growth retardation).

Breakout Point |
- Increased incidence with history of irradiation, NF-1, and p53 mutations (Li-Fraumeni syndrome)
- Range from pilocytic astrocytoma to malig-nant invasive anaplastic astrocytoma

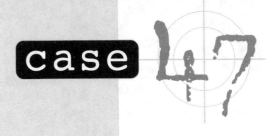

case 47

ID/CC A **66-year-old woman** presents to the clinic stating that the **taste and smell** of food has changed.

HPI She also noticed that over the past year, she has been having intermittent **frontal headaches**, and her **vision has deteriorated** significantly despite using reading glasses. She has no significant past medical history.

PE VS: normal. PE: funduscopic examination of left eye reveals a pale disc (due to **optic atrophy**) and right eye reveals **papilledema**. Intact taste sensation to salty, sweet, bitter, and sour. However, she is **unable to appreciate the smell** of peppermint, coffee, and cinnamon bilaterally.

Labs CBC, BMP, LFTs are all normal.

Imaging CT, head.

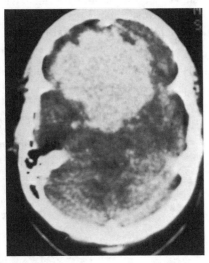

Figure 47-1. CT Head (noncontrast): large frontal hyperdense lesion.

case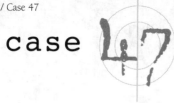

Meningioma

Pathogenesis

Meningiomas are slow-growing tumors that arise from the **arachnoidal cells** and can occur **intracranially** or in the **spinal canal.** They are usually **benign** and cause symptoms by compressing nearby structures depending on their location, such as **anosmia** when they compress the **olfactory bulbs** or tracts (which patients may describe as loss of taste). Vision also can be affected if the enlarging tumor encroaches on the optic nerves or chiasm.

Epidemiology

Meningiomas are found incidentally in 2.3% of autopsy cases. They constitute approximately 20% of all primary intracranial tumors, and 10% of meningiomas are located at the olfactory cribriform regions. The incidence increases with advancing age.

Management

Small **asymptomatic** meningiomas discovered incidentally do not need immediate treatment and can be **followed with serial head CT scans.** Larger symptomatic lesions require **surgical resection.**

Complications

Cerebral edema, visual disturbances.

Breakout Point

- Arises from dura mater or arachnoid
- Well-encapsulated, compress rather than invade, so surgically resectable
- Presents according to tumor site: unilateral proptosis, anosmia, optic nerve compression

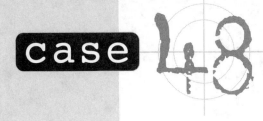
ID/CC	A **47-year-old man** complains of difficulty **hearing** in the right ear and difficulty with **balance** for the past 6 months.
HPI	He also complains of **tinnitus** and discomfort in the right ear and occasional **headache.**
PE	Mild **facial numbness** on the right side. Hearing is slightly decreased on the right when tested using a **512 Hz** tuning fork. Weber test: sound lateralizes to the left ear (opposite to ear with reduced hearing, suggesting sensorineural hearing loss). Rinne test: air conduction > bone conduction (ruling out conductive hearing loss).
Labs	Not applicable.
Investigations	**Audiometry: sensorineural pattern of hearing loss** with high-frequency pure-tone hearing and poor speech discrimination.
Imaging	MRI, brain.

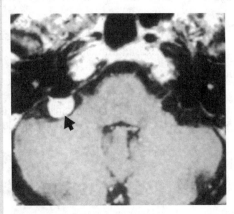

Figure 48-1. MRI, brain with contrast: an enhancing lesion around CN VIII on the right.

case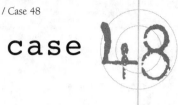

Acoustic Neuroma

Pathogenesis	Acoustic neuroma, also called acoustic **schwannoma**, is usually a **benign** encapsulated **slow-growing** tumor, which typically arises from the **Schwann cell sheath** of the **vestibular** portion of the acoustic nerve (CNVIII) at the cerebellopontine angle or in the internal auditory canal. As the tumor grows, it compresses or displaces cranial nerves, brain stem, or the cerebellum. Due to its proximity to the trigeminal nerve and facial nerve, symptoms related to dysfunction of these cranial nerves are common. Asymmetric sensorineural hearing loss is the hallmark of acoustic neuroma.
Epidemiology	Typically are isolated lesions in adults age 30 to 60. Bilateral acoustic neuromas are associated with **neurofibromatosis type 2,** which is autosomal recessive due to a defect on chromosome 22.
Management	Resection by **microsurgery; stereotactic radiosurgery.**
Complications	Obstruction of the CSF can cause hydrocephalus and increased intracranial pressure.
Breakout Point	• CNVIII schwannoma is present at the cerebellopontine angle • Bilateral and familial when associated with NF-2 • Presents with hearing loss; also tinnitus, headache

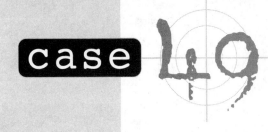

case **49**

ID/CC A **5-year-old boy** presents with **diabetes insipidus** and **vertical nystagmus**.

HPI He also complains of frequent **headaches**, and occasional **nausea** with the headaches. He also has a **shorter stature** compared to his brothers at the same age.

PE VS: normal. PE: short for age; papilledema and optic disk swelling (due to increased ICP) as well as **bitemporal hemianopsia** (due to impingement on optic chiasm).

Labs CBC: normal. Lytes: hypernatremia. UA: low specific gravity (<1.006) (due to diabetes insipidus).

Imaging CT, head: irregular mixed-density mass with small calcifications.

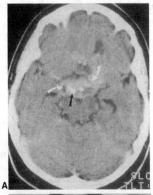

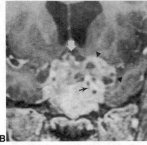

Figure 49-1. CT, head: Axial contrast-enhanced CT scan showed an irregular mixed-density mass with small calcifications. MRI, brain: enhancing **cystic, multilobulated suprasellar mass.**

97

case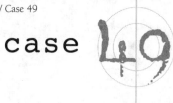

Craniopharyngioma

Pathogenesis

Craniopharyngioma is a slow-growing tumor that is embryologically derived from squamous cell **remnants of Rathke's pouch.** It usually arises in the pituitary stalk in the **suprasellar region** adjacent to the optic chiasm. Common symptoms include **pituitary hypofunction, visual difficulties,** and **severe headaches.** The clinical significance of this **histologically benign** tumor lies in its proximity to the optic chiasm, the carotid arteries, CN III, and the pituitary stalk.

Epidemiology

The **third most common intracranial tumor in children;** bimodal age distribution with a second peak in incidence in the fifth decade of life.

Management

Gross total surgical resection can be curative. However, gross total resection is not always possible due to the location of the tumor. Partial resection followed by radiotherapy or radiotherapy alone can achieve similar cure rate but with lower morbidity and mortality.

Complications

Necrosis of the pituitary stalk during surgery with release of ADH and a sharp decrease in urinary volume; postoperative recurrence of tumor, and pituitary hypofunction after treatment.

Breakout Point

- Derived from remnants of Rathke's pouch in the pituitary stalk in the suprasellar region compressing the optic chiasm
- Presents with endocrine dysfunction from pituitary involvement (hypothyroidism, adrenal insufficiency, diabetes insipidus)
- Presents with visual disturbance (bitemporal hemianopsia) from optic chiasm compression

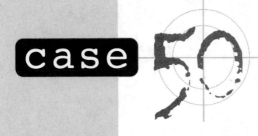

ID/CC	A **22-year-old woman** with **amenorrhea** and **headache**.
HPI	She also has **galactorrhea** and breast tenderness. Her headaches have been progressive with associated **photophobia.** She has unsuccessfully tried to conceive for 6 months.
PE	VS: normal. PE: well appearing. Optic discs have mild pallor (due to increased ICP), decreased peripheral vision (**bitemporal hemianopsia).**
Labs	CBC/Lytes: normal. TSH, LH, FSH: normal. **Increased prolactin.** ACTH stimulation test: normal.
Imaging	MRI, T1-coronal image of an anterior pituitary gland.

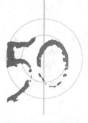

case 50

Pituitary Adenoma

Pathogenesis

Hyperpituitarism is most commonly caused by benign adenomas in the anterior pituitary. These small tumors can be functional or silent (about one-fifth). Functional adenomas are classified based on the hormones that they produce (this patient had a prolactinoma). Clinically, pituitary adenomas are classified as microadenomas (<1 cm) and macroadenomas (>1 cm). The clinical signs of pituitary adenomas are based on **endocrinologic disturbances** and **mass effects** as the adenoma fills the sella turcica and impinges on the nearby optic chiasm. In general, nonsecretory adenomas tend to be larger at the time of diagnosis than secretory adenomas.

Epidemiology

Pituitary adenomas comprise 10% of all intracranial neoplasia. One-third of pituitary adenomas are associated with multiple endocrine neoplasia (MEN-1), a familial disorder of endocrine tumors often involving the pituitary gland.

Management

Bromocriptine is a dopamine agonist used for prolactin and GH secreting adenomas. Radiation or gamma knife of pituitary gland is used for GH, ACTH, LH, FSH, TSH secreting adenomas. **Transsphenoidal surgery.**

Complications

Visual loss. Pituitary apoplexy (hemorrhage into the growing adenoma) can cause adrenal crisis and death. Nonsecretory adenomas can displace normal pituitary tissue, causing hypopituitarism.

Breakout Point

- Prolactinoma presents with amenorrhea, galactorrhea, infertility in women
- Prolactinoma presents with decreased libido, erectile dysfunction in men
- Can present with bitemporal hemianopsia (optic chiasm compression)

■ TABLE 50-1 ANTERIOR PITUITARY ADENOMAS

Hormone	Symptoms
Prolactin (PRL)	Women: Galactorrhea, Amenorrhea
	Men: Hypogonadism
TSH (Rare)	Thyrotoxicosis
GH	Before puberty: Gigantism
	After puberty: Acromegaly
ACTH	Cushing's Disease
FSH, LH	Rarely secretory
	Often detected because of neurologic disturbances

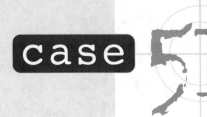

case 51

ID/CC A **9-year-old boy** presents with **headaches** and **difficulty walking.**

HPI He has had morning **headaches** with associated **nausea** and refractory **vomiting** for more than 2 months. He then developed an **unsteady gait** and ataxia over the last 2 weeks.

PE VS: normal. PE: neck supple; bilateral **papilledema;** abdomen benign; strength 5/5 throughout; **ataxic, wide-based gait;** extremity dysmetria.

Labs CBC/Lytes: normal. LFTs: normal. PT/PTT: normal. LP: no malignant cells.

Imaging CT, head: **midline cerebellar mass** with surrounding edema.

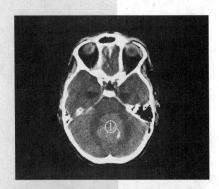

Figure 51-1. CT, head: **midline cerebellar mass** (1) with surrounding edema and enlarged ventricles.

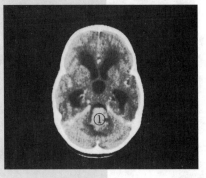

Figure 51-2. CT, head (with contrast): a different case with an enhancing cerebellar vermis mass (1) and obstructive hydrocephalus.

case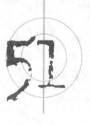

Medulloblastoma

Pathogenesis

Medulloblastoma is a highly malignant tumor that arises from neural precursor cells on the **floor of the fourth ventricle** and may block the flow of CSF, resulting in increased ICP and hydrocephalus.

Epidemiology

Infratentorial medulloblastomas are the most common malignant brain tumor in children, accounting for 80% of brain tumors diagnosed in children. The **male-to-female ratio** is **2:1**; 5-year survival is 50%.

Management

Surgery is performed to establish the diagnosis and debulk the tumor. **Radiotherapy** or chemotherapy is subsequently initiated.

Complications

Radiotherapy may lead to cognitive delay as well as to endocrine abnormalities. CSF dissemination and **metastasis** to meninges, spinal cord, and bone.

Breakout Point

- Most commonly presents in children in cerebellum (posterior fossa)
- Presents with truncal or gait ataxia

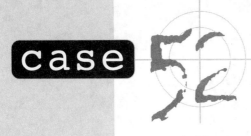

case 52

ID/CC   A **2-year-old girl** is brought to the ER by her parents, who have noticed her abdomen to be **full** and **distended.**

HPI   She is a healthy child who is up-to-date on her vaccinations. For the past week, her parents have noted a **left-sided abdominal mass.**

PE   VS: normal. PE: playful and in no acute distress; large, nontender left-sided abdominal mass with firm, irregular surface. The mass crosses the midline.

Labs   CBC: normal. UA: **elevated vanillylmandelic acid** (VMA is a catecholamine metabolite). Bone marrow biopsy is negative.

Imaging   U/S, abdomen: large left-sided abdominal mass. CT, chest and pelvis: normal. Bone scan: no bony metastases. MIBG (nuclear scan): increase uptake in the abdominal mass but no other sites of uptake.

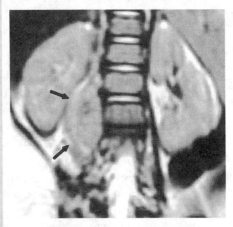

Figure 52-1. CT abdomen: Different patient with similar abdominal mass (*arrows*).

case 52

Neuroblastoma

Pathogenesis

Neuroblastoma **arises from primitive neural crest cells** that form the adrenal medulla and the cervical and thoracic sympathetic chains. It is characterized by defective catecholamine synthesis, which results in the accumulation and excretion of the intermediates homovanillic acid (HVA), VMA, and dopamine. N-*myc* oncogene amplification occurs in 20% of primary neuroblastoma tumors and is thought to contribute to its malignant potential.

Epidemiology

A common childhood tumor. Mean age of onset is 20 months. Two-thirds of cases occur within the **first 5 years of life.** About two-thirds of neuroblastomas originate in the **abdomen** and two-thirds of those originate in the **adrenal gland.**

Management

Staging workup includes bone marrow biopsy, bone radiographs, technetium radionuclide scan or MIBG scan, abdominal imaging by CT or MRI scan, and chest radiograph. A high rate of spontaneous regression is seen in infants with Stage 4s disease; these patients are generally observed and managed conservatively. In low risk and resectable disease, **surgical resection** with or without adjuvant chemotherapy is the mainstay of treatment. In unresectable disease, radiotherapy is used for local treatment followed by chemotherapy. In high-risk disease, surgical resection followed by radiotherapy and chemotherapy is the treatment of choice.

Complications

Complications include invasion of abdominal organs and **metastases** to **liver, lung,** and **bone.** Paraneoplastic syndromes include opsoclonus myoclonus (rapid, dancing eye movements, rhythmic jerking, or ataxia), and VIP secretion.

Breakout Point

- Small round blue cell neoplasm in Homer-Wright pseudorosettes
- Results in buildup of HVA, VMA, and dopamine (precursors of catecholamines)
- N-myc amplification

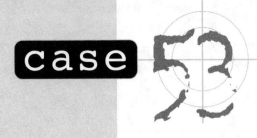

case

ID/CC   A **65-year-old man** who has been treated with **vincristine** for chronic lymphocytic leukemia complains of **tingling** (PARESTHESIAS) of the hands and feet and **constipation**.

HPI   The tingling began in his fingers 2 months ago after treatment with vincristine began; only recently has he experienced tingling in the toes. The sensation is constant and does not change with movement or position.

PE   VS: normal. PE: speech appropriate; cranial nerves intact; motor strength 5/5; DTRs 2+ except 1+ in Achilles (early loss of symmetrical ankle jerk); Babinski's sign absent; **decreased pinprick sensation from midfoot and wrists distally;** proprioception and vibration intact.

Labs   ESR, B_{12}, folate, TSH, hemoglobin A_{1C}, and serum protein electrophoresis normal; reduction in sensory nerve action potential.

Imaging   None.

case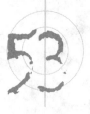

Peripheral Neuropathy Due to Vincristine

Pathogenesis

Vinca alkaloids such as vincristine function as **mitotic spindle inhibitors** and interact with tubulin, resulting in the impairment of axonal transport.

Epidemiology

Vincristine is the chemotherapeutic agent that is most commonly associated with **peripheral neuropathy.** Other common causes of drug-induced peripheral neuropathies include **cisplatin** (pure sensory neuropathy), **taxol, dapsone** (pure motor, resembles amyotrophic lateral sclerosis), **ethionamide, INH, hydralazine, phenytoin, Adriamycin,** and nucleoside analogs (antiretrovirals).

Management

Reduction or withdrawal of vincristine to allow remission of symptoms. If motor signs are present, the drug needs to be stopped. If some residual paresthesia remains, symptomatic treatment can be initiated with **gabapentin** or **amitriptyline.** Stool softeners and mild cathartics may be given at the beginning of treatment.

Complications

If not properly identified and if vincristine is not discontinued, the neuropathy will progress. This will result in eventual axonal damage, causing **motor weakness.** The sensory neuropathy will also worsen, extending further up the arms and legs. Acute **intestinal ileus** and **bladder neuropathies** (serious autonomic involvement) are two absolute contraindications to continued vincristine therapy.

Breakout Point

- Vincristine is the most common chemotherapeutic agent to cause peripheral neuropathy
- Most toxic neuropathies cause "dying back" axonal degeneration

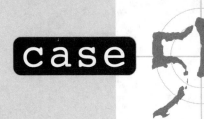

case 54

ID/CC A **45-year-old man** complains of slowly **progressive muscle weakness** involving the **hands and lower limbs.**

HPI He initially noticed reduced finger dexterity and wrist drop (EXTREMITY WEAKNESS), and his family noticed occasional slurring of words and choking at meals (BULBAR SIGNS). He has had muscle wasting, weakness, rigidity, and slowness. He denies any incontinence or changes in his bowel habits. He has also noted difficulty walking.

PE VS: normal. PE: **muscle atrophy,** weakness, wasting, **fasciculations,** loss of stretch reflexes, and bradykinesia noted in **upper extremities** bilaterally (LMN signs); **muscle rigidity, spasticity,** clonus, and hyperactive DTRs noted in bilateral **lower extremities** (UMN signs); **Babinski's sign present** (UMN sign); spastic gait; no sensory deficit; normal cognitive exam.

Labs Muscle biopsy shows **grouping of muscle fiber types** (as nerves die, adjacent nerves send buds to reinnervate muscle and fibers switch types). LP: mildly elevated protein (50 mg/dL) in CSF. EMG: **fasciculations** and evidence of **denervation** in upper extremities with **normal nerve conduction velocities.**

Imaging CT/MR, brain and spinal cord: normal.

case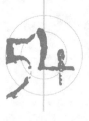

Amyotrophic Lateral Sclerosis

Pathogenesis | Amyotrophic lateral sclerosis (ALS), a.k.a. **Lou Gehrig's disease,** causes progressive muscle weakness and atrophy that typically begins distally and proceeds proximally. The cause is unknown, but glutamate toxicity, mitochondrial dysfunction, and autoimmunity may play a role. ALS affects both **anterior horn cells** in the spinal cord and **UMNs** in the corticospinal tract, resulting in both UMN and LMN deficits, which may be asymmetric.

Epidemiology | **Males** are more likely to be affected than females. **Incidence rises after age 40** and continues to increase until about 80. Occasionally associated with dementia and parkinsonism. A familial form of the disease with autosomal-dominant inheritance has been identified.

Management | **No specific treatment. Riluzole,** which reduces the presynaptic release of glutamate, may slow progression. Symptomatic management is indicated, including anticholinergics to prevent drooling and braces and physical therapy to assist mobility and prevent contractures.

Complications | Dysphagia, respiratory compromise, and aspiration; **death often within 5 years of symptom onset.**

Breakout Point |
- Both upper and lower motor neuron disease of the limbs
- SOD1 mutation in familial ALS

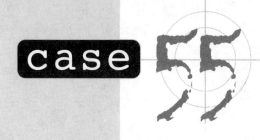

case **55**

ID/CC A **33-year-old woman** who **recently had a URI** now complains of **loss of strength in her lower legs** and unsteadiness when walking.

HPI Over the past 4 weeks, she has noted **symmetric weakness** with foot drop starting in her lower limbs and progressing to her hips and upper limbs (ASCENDING PARALYSIS). Over the past week, she has experienced occasional urinary retention, lightheadedness on rising quickly, and shortness of breath.

PE VS: no fever; **orthostatic hypotension; tachycardia** (due to autonomic dysfunction). PE: mental status normal; marked symmetric **loss of motor strength** with **flaccidity** most notable in **proximal lower limbs; absent patellar and Achilles reflexes bilaterally** (AREFLEXIA); mild facial weakness.

Labs LP: **elevated protein in CSF; normal cellularity** (CYTOALBUMINIC DISSOCIATION). Serum B_{12} normal; FTA-ABS negative; glucose normal. Lytes: normal. EMG: markedly slowed motor and sensory conduction. Nerve conduction studies reveal evidence of **demyelination** with **slowing of conduction velocity** and multifocal conduction blocks.

Imaging CT/MR, brain: no intracranial lesions or hemorrhage.

PERIPHERAL NERVE

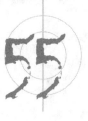

case 55

Guillain–Barré Syndrome

Pathogenesis

Guillain–Barré syndrome is an acute demyelinating polyradiculoneuropathy that is believed to be an **autoimmune-mediated reaction** to certain infectious agents. Progressive ascending flaccid paralysis peaks within 4 weeks of onset. The most common pathogens are thought to be *Campylobacter jejuni*, viral hepatitis, and EBV. Guillain–Barré syndrome can also occur following influenza vaccinations.

Epidemiology

There is a bimodal age distribution, with most cases occurring in early adulthood or between 45 and 64 years. There is no known HLA association.

Management

Plasmapheresis is the treatment of choice. Patients with hemodynamic instability and children may be given **IVIG.** Hospitalization for potential respiratory failure (and subsequent mechanical ventilation).

Complications

Resulting **respiratory insufficiency** may require ventilatory support. Approximately 85% of patients make a complete or nearly complete recovery, with the mortality rate standing at 3 to 4%. Mortality arises from cardiac arrhythmias or superimposed viral or bacterial pneumonia.

Breakout Point

- Classically preceded by *Campylobacter jejuni* gastroenteritis or URI (1 to 3 weeks prior)
- Symmetric, bilateral, ascending weakness with areflexia
- Cytoalbuminemic dissociation in CSF: high protein but no or few WBC

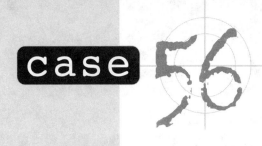

case 56

ID/CC   A **5-year-old Amish boy** presents with a 3-day history of progressive **leg weakness.**

HPI   He has **not had any immunizations.** He began having muscle pain and spasms 3 days ago; weakness has progressed such that he is now unable to climb stairs. He also complains of tingling in the legs but denies any weakness in his arms or any prior trauma.

PE   VS: fever (38.3°C); normal BP. PE: alert and oriented; CN II–XII intact; motor tone normal in both arms but **flaccid in both legs; motor strength 3/5** in both legs; **DTRs absent bilaterally** in patella and Achilles; **sensory exam intact** to all primary modalities; sphincter tone normal. On follow-up exam 3 weeks later, lower extremity muscular atrophy is apparent (and remains permanent).

Labs   CBC: normal. LP: CSF cultures positive for poliovirus. Throat and stool cultures positive; PCR positive for poliovirus anti-RNA.

Imaging   None.

case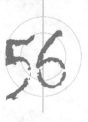

Poliomyelitis

Pathogenesis

The causative agent of poliomyelitis is **poliovirus** serotypes 1, 2, and 3. The enterovirus (picornavirus family) **enters the body via the GI tract** and multiplies in the lymphoid tissue of the GI tract; it then spreads to the CNS via the bloodstream, where it attacks the **motor neurons of the spinal cord** and **brain stem.** Person-to-person spread is via the oral–oral or oral–fecal route.

Epidemiology

Because of effective mass immunization, the annual incidence of polio in the United States has markedly decreased. Outbreaks occur in low-vaccination communities (such as the Amish) and in those exposed to wild-type polio virus type I.

Management

Prevention with immunization is essential. Bed rest during the first few days reduces the risk of paralysis. Airway maintenance and ventilatory support as necessary. No specific treatment.

Complications

Autonomic instability resulting in cardiac arrhythmias and wide variation in blood pressure. Bulbar polio may jeopardize respiratory center function.

Breakout Point

- Polio virus infection of the anterior horn motor neurons of the spinal cord and brain stem
- Presents with flaccid, asymmetric weakness
- Leads to muscle atrophy

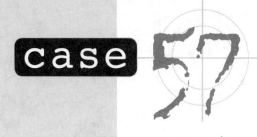
PERIPHERAL NERVE

ID/CC A **43-year-old right-handed** administrative assistant **(woman)** presents with 6 months of **tingling** and **numbness** in her **thumb, index finger,** and **middle finger** on the **right**.

HPI The sensory symptoms are worst at night and when she first wakes up in the morning. She complains of **mild right hand weakness,** particularly with opening jars. She has no pain in her neck and has noted no disturbances of her speech or language.

PE VS: normal. PE: sensation to pain and temperature are decreased over the palmar surface of the thumb, index finger, middle finger, and the radial half of the ring finger in the right hand. There is mild weakness of abductor pollicis brevis and mild atrophy of the thenar eminence in the right hand, but strength in the other muscles is normal. Percussion over the anterior wrist consistently reproduces a shooting paresthesia from the wrist to palm and first three fingers (POSITIVE TINEL'S TEST). Forced flexion at the wrists (PHALEN'S TEST) produces discomfort and tingling in the right wrist.

Labs CBC, chemistry panel, LFTs, TFTs, and B_{12} levels are all normal. EMG: **slowed conduction velocity** in the **median nerve** across the right wrist.

Imaging None.

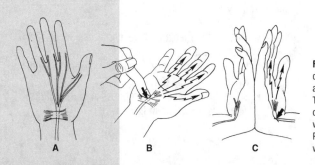

Figure 57-1. (A) Normal distribution of the median nerve. **(B)** Eliciting Tinel's sign by percussing over the anterior wrist. **(C)** Eliciting Phalen's sign by holding wrists in extreme flexion.

113

case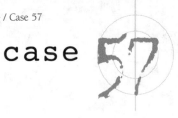

Carpal Tunnel Syndrome

Pathogenesis

Carpal tunnel syndrome (CTS) is a mononeuropathy caused by **compression** of the **median nerve** at the **wrist**, under the **flexor retinaculum**. It is characterized by numbness and paresthesias in the distribution of the median nerve in the fingers, but spares the palm, because the sensory branch to the palm arises proximal to the carpal tunnel. Sensory deficit in the **fourth digit** is limited to the **radial half** of the finger as the ulnar nerve supplies the ulnar half of the digit. Medical conditions that cause fluid retention or inflammation and predispose to CTS include hypothyroidism, rheumatoid arthritis, and pregnancy. The dominant hand tends to be affected earlier and to a greater extent than the nondominant hand.

Epidemiology

CTS is very common with increased incidence in women and those with advanced age and a history of trauma. Manual labor and computer work also hasten development of CTS.

Management

Conservative management with rest, wrist splints (especially at night), and modification of the work environment. Local corticosteroid injections may be effective. Surgical resection of the transverse carpal ligament to release the entrapped median nerve in refractory cases.

Complications

Progressive weakness and atrophy of the muscles supplied by the median nerve.

Breakout Point

- Caused by median nerve compression at the anterior wrist
- Tinel's sign: paresthesia elicited by percussing wrist over carpal tunnel
- Phalen's sign: painful numbness in thumb/digits with holding wrists in flexion

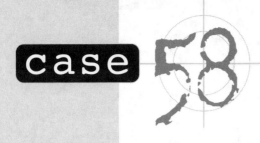case 58

ID/CC A **76-year-old woman** presents with **imbalance** and fatigue.

HPI She has overall **weakness, anorexia** with a 10-lb. weight loss and a burning sensation in her tongue (**glossitis**).

PE VS: normal. PE: **elderly woman** with pallor and mild **icterus; bilateral weakness** and **decreased positional** sense in her legs > arms; **lower extremity reflexes** decreased; Romberg sign present with **ataxia.**

Labs CBC with PBS: anemia (Hb 9), MCV 107 (**macro-ovalocytes**), **high RDW, hypersegmented neutrophils; increased indirect bilirubin** and **LDH;** decreased serum cobalamin; antibodies to intrinsic factor present (**Schilling Test** or serological testing) and low levels of gastric acid (**achlorhydria).**

Imaging None.

case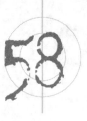

Vitamin B$_{12}$ Deficiency

Pathogenesis

Decreased absorption of vitamin B$_{12}$ occurs through multiple mechanisms, but commonly is caused by **pernicious anemia**. This results from auto-antibodies to intrinsic factor (IF) and the gastric parietal cell that produces IF (**atrophic gastritis**). IF is necessary to bind B$_{12}$ and facilitate ileal absorption. Other causes of B$_{12}$ deficiency include inadequate diet (vegan), inadequate absorption (Crohn's, Sprue, bacterial overgrowth in a blind loop of the intestine), inadequate utilization, increased requirements (tapeworms), and increased excretion. Neurologic degenerative "combined system disease" involves both the central white matter and peripheral nerves, both sensory and motor. Symptoms begin as vibrational and sensory in the lower extremities and progress to spasticity, Babinski responses, and "megaloblastic mania" (paranoia, delirium, confusion). The posterior columns and corticospinal tracts are affected in late stages.

Epidemiology

There are multiple pathways that result in low levels of vitamin B$_{12}$ (cobalamin). It often occurs in the fifth to eighth decades of life, more often in Western societies. Use of the Schilling test can help determine if poor absorption is the cause.

Management

Intramuscular vitamin B$_{12}$ supplementation for life unless the underlying mechanism is corrected; high dose oral vitamin B$_{12}$ (rarely used); do not give folic acid (instead of B$_{12}$) to patient with documented B$_{12}$ deficiency; may cause fulminant neurological sequelae.

Complications

Neurologic deficits can be irreversible. Increased risk for gastric cancer in pernicious anemia patients.

Breakout Point

- Triad of Heme, Neuro, GI symptoms
- Heme: megaloblastic anemia, oval macrocytes, hypersegmented neutrophils, lemon-yellow skin pallor, fatigue
- Neuro: numbness/tingling in lower extremities, loss of vibration and position sense, gait abnormalities, depression, dementia
- GI: beefy red tongue, diarrhea, constipation

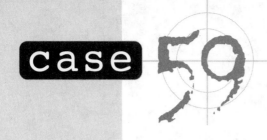

case 59

ID/CC	A **17-year-old man** who was **stabbed in the back** presents with **inability to use his left leg** along with stiffness and **loss of pain sensation in the right leg**.
HPI	The stab wound extended to the spinal cord at the level of L1 slightly to the left of the spinous process. Since the injury, the patient has been unable to move his left leg. He also complains of episodes of "tingling" of the distal left leg.
PE	VS: normal. PE: cranial nerves intact; motor exam demonstrates 5/5 strength bilaterally in upper extremities, 5/5 strength in right lower extremity, and 0/5 strength in left lower extremity; increased tone in left leg; DTRs 2+ and symmetric in upper extremities, 3+ in left patella and Achilles, and 2+ in right patella and Achilles; **diminished proprioception and vibration sense** in left leg; **loss of pain and temperature** sense in right leg; Babinski's sign present in left leg.
Labs	None.
Imaging	MR, spine: no intramedullary mass identified.

case 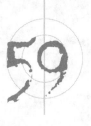 59

Brown-Séquard Syndrome

Pathogenesis	Brown-Séquard syndrome is due to **hemisection of the spinal cord.** This results in ipsilateral UMN signs below the lesion (hyperreflexia, spastic paralysis resulting from lateral corticospinal tract interruption), ipsilateral loss of vibration and proprioception sense (due to damage to the dorsal column), and contralateral loss of pain and temperature sensation (due to damage of the spinothalamic tract that decussated below the lesion).
Epidemiology	Typically occurs secondary to **trauma** (e.g., bullet or stab wounds), spinal cord **tumor,** or fracture-dislocation causing compression.
Management	**Symptomatic relief** of hyperesthesias; phenytoin and carbamazepine are effective.
Complications	Limited mobility may result in pressure ulcers or URIs; the neurologic syndrome itself does not progress.
Breakout Point	• Unilateral hemisection of the spinal cord • Presents with ipsilateral weak leg with brisk reflexes and contralateral strong leg with loss of pain and temperature sensation

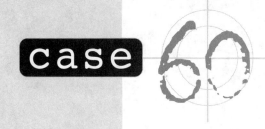

case 60

ID/CC	A **32-year-old man** fell two stories from the roof of a house and is now **unable to get up or move his legs**.
HPI	The patient was previously healthy.
PE	VS: normal. PE: able to follow commands; speech appropriate; cranial nerves intact; 5/5 strength in upper extremities; **0/5 motor strength in lower extremities;** DTRs 2+ in upper extremities; DTRs absent in lower extremities (may increase later); **no sensation to pinprick below iliac crest** (T12 sensory level); **rectal tone markedly diminished.**
Labs	None.
Imaging	MR, spine: fracture-dislocation of the T12 vertebral body with compression of the spinal cord (the majority of thoracolumbar fractures occur between T12 and L2).

SPINAL

case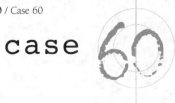

Spinal Cord Injury

Pathogenesis

There are **four types** of spinal injuries: flexion, extension, axial due to compressive force, and rotational. Spinal cord injury can result in neurogenic shock, when the sympathetic innervation to the vasculature is compromised; patients experience hypotension and bradycardia.

Epidemiology

Younger men are at highest risk. Associated with a mortality rate of 5 to 20%; quadriplegia is the end result in 30 to 40% of cases.

Management

ABCs; **mechanical** stabilization of the entire spine to prevent further injury. Insertion of nasogastric tube. Administer **IV methylprednisolone** within 24 hours of injury to minimize edema. **Surgery** to permanently stabilize the spine; intermittent straight catheterization for urinary incontinence. Baclofen for muscle spasms.

Complications

Autonomic dysfunction, respiratory and skin infections due to immobility, urinary incontinence, UTIs, painful muscle spasms, and constipation requiring daily bowel regimen (stool softener, enemas).

Breakout Point

- Acute loss of motor, sensory, autonomic, reflex function below level of lesion

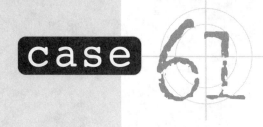

case 61

ID/CC A **51-year-old man** presents with **severe interscapular back pain, difficulty walking** for 1 week, and **urinary incontinence** over the past day.

HPI He has had **pain radiating** from his **mid-back to his torso** for 2 months. He also has **decreased appetite** and **weight loss** of 20 pounds over 1 month. There is no history of trauma or fever.

PE VS: normal. PE: tenderness to palpation in the upper back between the scapula. Mild **weakness** in the lower extremities bilaterally, with **increased tone, hyperreflexia,** and **Babinski signs present** bilaterally. Sensation to pain and temperature are decreased below a **sensory level at T6.** Joint position sense is absent in the lower extremities. **Rectal tone** is significantly **decreased,** and the post void residual is 500 cc (overflow incontinence).

Labs CBC/Lytes: normal. Prostate-specific antigen is 358 ng/mL.

Imaging MRI, spine: mass lesion compressing the spinal cord in the mid-thoracic spine.

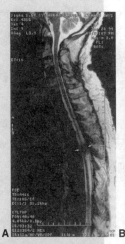
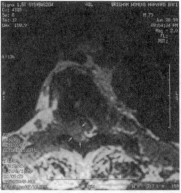

Figure 61-1. MRI, spine: mass lesion compressing the spinal cord in the mid-thoracic spine.

SPINAL

121

case 61

Spinal Cord Compression (From Metastatic Prostate Cancer)

Pathogenesis

Epidural spinal cord compression is a **neurologic emergency** that requires evaluation in **all** patients with a history of cancer who have back pain, leg weakness, or urinary/fecal incontinence. The most common tumors associated with cord compression are lung, breast, and prostate. The most common location for hematogenous spread of metastases is the thoracic spine. This patient demonstrates multiple upper neuron signs, including **spasticity, hyperreflexia, Babinski signs, lower extremity weakness, decreased rectal tone, urinary retention,** and a **sensory level**. Emergent imaging of the entire neuro-axis with MRI is indicated for all patients suspected of having the disorder, as metastases are frequently multiple. Prognosis depends on the severity of the deficit at initial diagnosis, e.g., most patients who present as ambulatory and receive treatment maintain the ability to ambulate. Overall, however, spinal cord compression portends a poor prognosis.

Epidemiology

Metastatic lesions in the spinal cord occur in approximately 5 to 10% of cancer patients.

Management

Give **corticosteroids** (e.g., dexamethasone 10 mg IV as a single bolus, followed by 4 mg every 6 hours) immediately if clinical suspicion is high. Perform **radiation therapy** as soon as possible. **Emergent surgical decompressive laminectomy** may be indicated in those with potential spinal instability or spinal cord compression due to bony disease, particularly in those who present with an acute onset of neurologic dysfunction.

Complications

Paraplegia or quadriplegia, depending on the level of spinal cord compression. Other persistent deficits include urinary dysfunction and loss of bowel continence.

Breakout Point

- Suspect in patients with cancer with new onset back pain
- Neurologic emergency
- Start steroids as early as possible

case 62

ID/CC A **62-year-old right-handed woman** with a history of **paroxysmal atrial tachycardia** is brought to the hospital after "not making sense" at work.

HPI The patient was at a meeting when she suddenly began **speaking "gibberish."** She was **unable to follow instructions** to rise from her chair. However, once her colleague helped her up, she was able to walk to the car without assistance.

PE VS: **hypertension** (BP 160/100); **pulse irregularly irregular.** PE: alert and in no acute distress with clear but unintelligible speech (FLUENT APHASIA); **unable to repeat phrases** or follow commands; **paraphasic errors** (e.g., "shoon" instead of "spoon") and **neologisms** (nonexistent words, e.g., "zork"); cranial nerves intact; motor strength 5/5 and DTRs 2+ throughout; Babinski's sign absent.

Labs CBC: normal. ECG: atrial fibrillation with controlled ventricular rate. Lytes: normal. PT/PTT and glucose normal.

Imaging CT, head (on admission): no mass; no hemorrhage; no infarct. CT, head (24 hours after admission): ischemic infarct in the left superior temporal gyrus. US, carotid: no hemodynamically significant stenosis. Echo: dilated left atrium; no thrombus.

case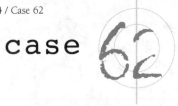

Wernicke's Aphasia

Pathogenesis	Wernicke's aphasia is typically due to a **cardioembolic event**. Patients are often unaware that their speech is incomprehensible.
Epidemiology	The annual risk of stroke with atrial fibrillation is 5%.
Management	The patient's age, the size of the stroke, and the status of the unaffected hemisphere determine the level of recovery from the aphasia. To prevent recurrent strokes, place patients with atrial fibrillation on **lifelong anticoagulation** with **warfarin** or **antiplatelet** agents. Speech therapy is useful.
Complications	Recurrent stroke and MI.
Breakout Point	

- **Wernicke's aphasia is Wordy** but makes no sense (receptive aphasia)
- Do not confuse with Wernicke encephalopathy, which is due to thiamine deficiency

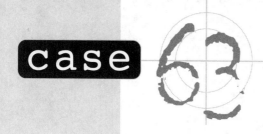

case 63

ID/CC A **62-year-old right-handed man** with a history of hypertension and tobacco use presents with an acute onset **inability to speak.**

HPI He was well this morning, but during a meeting his speech became slow and then stopped altogether. He was **able to follow instructions** to get up and walk but needed help walking. He was brought to the ER by a colleague. The patient has a history of **hypercholesterolemia.**

PE VS: normal HR; hypertension (BP 185/95). PE: alert and **able to follow commands** but **unable to repeat commands; nonfluent speech;** able to name two of three objects but unable to name parts of objects; right facial droop; right upper extremity 3/5, and right lower extremity 4/5 on motor exam.

Labs CBC/Lytes: normal. PT/PTT and glucose normal. ECG: sinus rhythm with LVH.

Imaging CT, brain (on admission): no hemorrhage; no mass; no shift. CT, brain (24 hours later): ischemic **infarct of the left posterior inferior frontal gyrus** (BROCA'S AREA). US, carotid: 80% left **ICA stenosis.** Echo: no thrombus.

case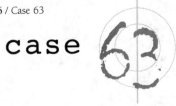

Broca's Aphasia

Pathogenesis	Broca's aphasia is a nonfluent (motor) aphasia characterized by broken speech in which patients are unable to produce spoken language, but **comprehension** of speech **remains intact.** Characteristically, patients are aware of their deficit and are frustrated with their inability to communicate. Hypertension, **diabetes,** cardiac disease, AIDS, drug abuse, heavy alcohol consumption, elevated serum cholesterol, and tobacco use are independent risk factors for the development of ischemic stroke.
Epidemiology	An estimated 500,000 new cases of stroke of all types occur each year; strokes are a common cause of death and disability. Modifiable risk factors include tobacco use, hypertension, diabetes mellitus, and hypercholesterolemia.
Management	**Antiplatelet agent** (e.g., aspirin) for secondary stroke prevention; heparin for DVT prophylaxis. Hold antihypertensive agents for 2 to 4 weeks, as cerebral hypoperfusion is a risk. Six weeks after stroke, obtain an MR to confirm the extent of ICA stenosis. **Carotid endarterectomy** is indicated if stenosis on symptomatic side is >70%. Endarterectomy is not indicated until 6 weeks after acute stroke.
Complications	Recurrent ischemic infarcts and CAD. Depression can also occur, because patients are aware of their deficit.
Breakout Point	• BROca's aphasia produces BROken speech (expressive aphasia)

ID/CC A **57-year-old left-handed African-American man** complains of acute-onset, **severe headache** and then develops **weakness on the left side of his body** (HEMIPLEGIA).

HPI He has **hypertension** that has been treated with multiple antihypertensives. Three months ago, he stopped taking all his prescription medications (NONCOMPLIANT). He was asymptomatic until this morning.

PE VS: **hypertension** (BP 205/110); normal HR. PE: lethargic; responsive to voices but unable to follow commands; positive **doll's eyes;** left **facial droop** but able to raise eyebrows (UPPER MOTOR NEURON LEFT FACIAL PALSY); motor strength 0/5 in left upper and lower extremity; left Babinski's sign present.

Labs CBC/Lytes: normal. Glucose normal, PT/PTT and platelets normal. ECG: sinus rhythm with LVH.

Imaging CT, head: focal hemorrhage involving the right basal ganglia.

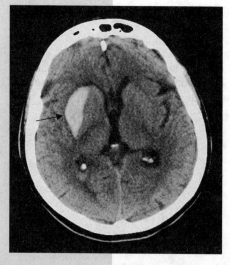

Figure 64-1. CT, head (noncontrast): focal hemorrhage involving the right basal ganglia.

case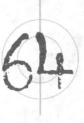

Stroke, Hypertensive

Pathogenesis

The **most common causes** of intracerebral hemorrhage are **hypertension, vascular malformation, tumor,** and **cerebral amyloid angiopathy**. The most common sites of hypertensive hemorrhage are the basal ganglia (putamen and thalamus), cerebellum, and pons.

Epidemiology

Fifteen percent of all strokes are hemorrhagic. Up to 60% of hemorrhagic strokes are due to hypertension.

Management

Intubate for airway protection; administer **IV beta-blockers to keep systolic BP <150** (reduce blood pressure to the lowest level that can maintain cerebral perfusion). Mechanical hyperventilation and IV mannitol can be used if ICP is increased. These treatments will stabilize the patient in preparation for surgical intervention to prevent brain stem herniation.

Complications

Recurrent stroke and hypertensive encephalopathy. Early mortality rate is higher than observed in infarction. Level of consciousness is a strong prognostic factor. Comatose patients have a mortality rate of approximately 90%.

Breakout Point

- Hypertension is a major risk factor for both hemorrhagic and ischemic stroke
- Intracerebral hemorrhage is indistinguishable clinically from ischemic stroke but causes increased ICP and higher risk of seizure

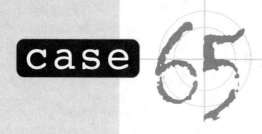

ID/CC A **44-year-old woman** presents to the ER with the **worst headache of her life,** which began 1 week ago but has grown intense over the past few hours.

HPI She also had **nausea, vomiting, neck stiffness, and photophobia.** While in the ER, she lost consciousness. On arousal, she developed a **right facial droop** and **right hemiparesis.**

PE VS: tachycardia (HR 112); slight fever (37.8 C) PE: moaning, irritable, and confused; **decerebrate posturing;** depressed level of consciousness; **nuchal rigidity; Kernig's and Brudzinski's signs positive left facial droop; left hemiplegia; left hyperreflexia;** fundoscopy reveals **papilledema.** No other focal neurological signs noted.

Labs CBC: normal. Lytes: hyponatremia (due to SIADH). PT/PTT normal (rules out SAH due to blood dyscrasias). LP: not done, since CT confirmed diagnosis. (CSF would have been **grossly bloody** with a **xanthochromic appearance** to the centrifuged supernatant.)

Imaging CT, head: hyperdensity within the left sylvian, anterior interhemispheric, and quadrigeminal cisterns.

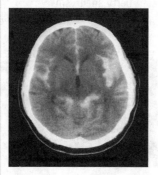

Figure 65-1. CT, head (noncontrast): hyperdensity within the left sylvian, anterior interhemispheric, and quadrigeminal cisterns.

case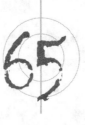

Subarachnoid Hemorrhage

Pathogenesis

Subarachnoid hemorrhage may be heralded by **a pro-dromal phase** with a sentinel headache that precedes the hemorrhagic event. The most common cranial nerve palsy is that of the **oculomotor nerve.** Associated signs of meningeal irritation **(meningismus)** are often seen.

Epidemiology

Shows slight female predominance.

Management

Surgical clipping; aneurysm coiling; blood pressure control. **Nimodipine,** a calcium channel blocker previously thought to prevent vasospasm, but now is thought to be neuroprotective in case of vasospasm. **Control of vasospasm:** includes HHH therapy (**H**ypertension, **H**ypervolemia, and **H**emodilution) to improve perfusion in the areas affected by the arterial spasm.

Complications

Rebleeding (risk highest in the first 48 hours), vasospasm, cerebral edema, hydrocephalus, SIADH, cerebral salt wasting (increased atrial natriuretic peptide).

Breakout Point

- Most common cause of spontaneous SAH is berry aneurysm
- Presents as "worst headache of my life"

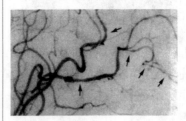

Figure 65-2. Cerebral angiogram: multiple areas of narrowing, representing vasospasm, which is the most common cause of death following SAH. It can occur 4 to 14 days post SAH.

ID/CC A **91-year-old right-handed woman** is found on the floor **unable to speak or move the right side of her body.**

HPI The patient lives alone and was last seen 2 days ago. The woman was grunting and not moving her right side.

PE VS: **hypotension** (BP 80/50); **irregularly irregular pulse** (due to atrial fibrillation; average HR 110). PE: alert; unable to speak spontaneously or to repeat or follow commands; motor strength 0/5 in right arm and leg with Babinski's sign present; reflexes 2+ and symmetric; no cranial nerve palsies.

Labs CBC normal. Elevated BUN (55 mg/dL); normal creatinine (1.1 mg/dL) (prerenal azotemia due to dehydration or low cardiac output). Lytes: normal. ECG: **atrial fibrillation** with fast ventricular rate.

Imaging CT, head: hypodensity involving the entire left MCA distribution (classic sign of completed ischemic infarct). Echo: no thrombus; dilated left atrium; LV ejection fraction of 55%.

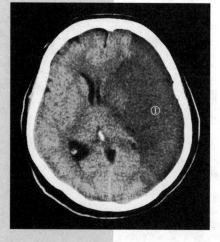

Figure 66-1. CT, head: hypodensity (1) involving the entire left MCA distribution (classic sign of completed ischemic infarct).

case 66

Stroke, Left MCA Infarct

Pathogenesis

Left MCA occlusion causes **contralateral hemiplegia, hemisensory loss,** and **loss of right visual field** (HOMONYMOUS HEMIANOPSIA). The inability to speak, repeat, and understand language (GLOBAL APHASIA) results when the dominant hemisphere is involved, including Broca's area, Wernicke's area, and the arcuate fasciculus. Left MCA infarction also causes aphasia, alexia, agraphia, acalculia, and right/left confusion in addition to right-sided hemiplegia.

Epidemiology

The annual risk of stroke with atrial fibrillation is 5%.

Management

Prevent recurrent strokes in those with atrial fibrillation by placing on **long-term anticoagulation with warfarin.** For maximal recovery after this event, physical, occupational, and speech therapy are necessary.

Complications

The most common complications are pneumonia and UTI due to Foley catheterization. Other complications include hemorrhagic transformation of the ischemic infarct and recurrent infarcts.

Breakout Point

- MCA is the most common vessel affected by stroke
- Due to homunculus, arm and face may be affected more than leg
- Contralateral hemiplegia, hemisensory, homonymous hemianopsia

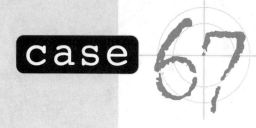

case 67

ID/CC	A **55-year-old right-handed woman** with **chronic hypertension** presents with **acute-onset left-sided weakness** and **altered sensorium**.
HPI	The patient is being treated for hypertension. This morning, her husband found her on the floor next to the bed, unable to move her left arm and leg. She could speak but was "acting funny."
PE	VS: **hypertension** (BP 180/100). PE: alert with fluent speech; answers questions appropriately but is **unable to draw a clock or copy a five-sided figure correctly; eyes deviated to right;** sensation absent to pinprick in left arm and leg; **0/5 strength in left arm and leg** and 5/5 strength in right arm and leg; DTRs 2+ in right arm and leg and 3+ in left arm and leg; increased tone in left arm and leg, normal in right arm and leg; Babinski's sign present on left; no carotid or subclavian bruit; no cardiac murmurs.
Labs	CBC/Lytes: normal. PT/PTT and glucose normal. VDRL negative; antiphospholipid antibodies negative; elevated cholesterol and triglycerides.
Imaging	CT, head (within 24 hours): no mass, hemorrhage, or midline shift. CT, head (after 48 hours): right MCA infarct with extensive hypodensity.

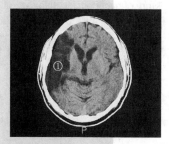

Figure 67-1. CT, head (after 48 hours): right MCA infarct with extensive hypodensity (1).

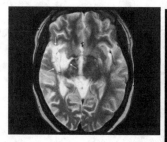

Figure 67-2. MR, brain: another patient with a smaller T2-hyper-intense right MCA infarct.

STROKE

case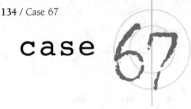

Stroke, Right MCA Infarct

Pathogenesis

Hypertension is an independent risk factor for the development of ischemic stroke. Right MCA occlusion causes **contralateral hemiplegia, hemisensory loss,** spatial agnosia, and **loss of left visual field** (HOMONYMOUS HEMIANOPIA) with **deviation of the eyes to the side of the lesion.** There is also global aphasia if the dominant hemisphere is affected.

Epidemiology

There are 500,000 new strokes each year in the United States. Strokes are a common cause of disability. Modifiable risk factors include **tobacco use, hypertension, diabetes mellitus,** and **hypercholesterolemia.**

Management

Avoid a precipitous fall in blood pressure in order to maintain adequate cerebral perfusion. **Antiplatelet agents** reduce stroke risk by 25%; begin them after the initial head CT has ruled out cerebral hemorrhage. **Lipid-lowering drugs** also reduce the risk of recurrent stroke.

Complications

Complications include recurrent stroke, MI, DVT, UTI, and aspiration pneumonia. Loss of consciousness renders a poorer prognosis.

Breakout Point

- Strokes present with sudden onset of neurologic defect
- Associated with history of hypertension, hypercholesterolemia, diabetes mellitus, peripheral vascular disease

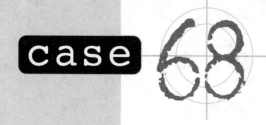

case 68

ID/CC	A **30-year-old man** presents with acute, severe onset of feeling "as if the **room was spinning**" (VERTIGO) and became nauseous and **vomited.** He had **pain and numbness** on the **right** side of his **face** (IPSILATERAL FACIAL PAIN AND NUMBNESS). He also noted **difficulty with swallowing** (DYSPHAGIA) and a **hoarse voice.**
HPI	When he attempted to stand and walk, he felt "as though I was being **pushed to the right,**" (LATEROPUL-SION) and **fell to the right** (IPSILATERAL ATAXIA). When he washed his hands in the sink, he **could not feel the temperature** of the water in his **left hand** but was able to sense pain and temperature on the right (CONTRALATERAL PAIN AND THERMAL SENSATION LOSS).
PE	VS: hypertensive (BP 160/100). PE: **nystagmus** in all directions of gaze, worst with right lateral gaze. Right eye: eyelid **ptosis,** R pupil diameter < L pupil diameter but both reactive, anhidrosis (IPSILATERAL HORNER'S SYNDROME). **Decreased sensation** on right side of face and left side of body. **CN IX and X:** Palate elevates poorly on the right; gag reflex absent on the right. Gait veers to right side.
Labs	CBC/Lytes: normal. PT/PTT normal.
Imaging	MRI, brain: T2 weighted axial image shows an infarct in the lateral right medulla in the distribution of the PICA artery.

STROKE

case 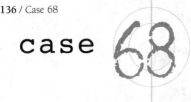 68

Wallenberg Syndrome (Lateral Medullary Infarct or PICA Syndrome)

Pathogenesis	Wallenberg syndrome is a brain stem infarction of the **lateral medulla** that may result from progression of **vertebrobasilar insufficiency** and compromise of the posterior inferior cerebellar artery (**PICA**). A stroke may occur by occlusion of the vertebral artery or its branches or emboli may travel distally. Symptoms of Wallenberg syndrome may persist for years.
Epidemiology	Risk factors include neck manipulation (trauma), connective tissue diseases such as Ehlers–Danlos syndrome, and stroke risk factors such as age, male sex, smoking, hypertension, and hypercholesterolemia.
Management	Supportive care. Avoid hypotension.
Complications	Aspiration pneumonia, compromise of the respiratory control centers in the brain stem (Ondine's curse), autonomic dysfunction (arrhythmias, GI distress).
Breakout Point	

Clinical Symptom or Sign	Neuroanatomic Lesion
Contralateral loss in pain and temperature from body	Lateral spinothalamic tract
Ipsilateral loss of pain and temperature from face	Spinal trigeminal nucleus
Ipsilateral dysphagia, hoarseness, diminished gag reflex	Nucleus ambiguus (CN IX and X)
Vertigo, diplopia, nystagmus, vomiting	Vestibular nuclei
Ipsilateral Horner's syndrome	Descending sympathetic fibers

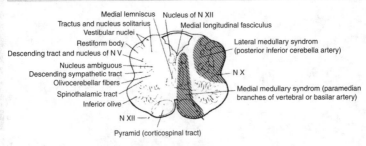

Figure 68-1. Lateral and Medial Medullary Syndromes.

ID/CC A **65-year-old man** presents with **sudden onset left eye blindness.** He states the vision in his left eye **painlessly turned to black, "as though a curtain was falling down."** His vision returned 10 minutes later.

HPI When he closed the right eye he could see nothing; when he closed the left eye his vision was intact. Three weeks ago, he recalls several minutes of **right arm and leg weakness** (recent TIA). He denies headache, history of migraine, fever, weight loss, or jaw claudication. He has a history of diabetes mellitus, hypertension, hypercholesterolemia, and a 45-pack-year history of smoking.

PE VS: normal. PE: visual acuity normal; fundoscopy reveals a **bright orange plaque** (HOLLENHURST PLAQUE) **in a retinal arteriole and a pale retina.** Left **carotid bruit.** No cardiac murmurs. Neurological exam noncontributory.

Labs CBC: normal. ESR normal. Coags normal.

Imaging US carotid: left internal carotid artery stenosis of 70 to 79%, right carotid artery has <40% stenosis. TTE: no source of thrombus. MRI/A, brain: no acute stroke, some periventricular white matter disease, normal intracranial vasculature.

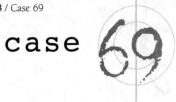

case 69

Stroke, Transient Monocular Blindness

Pathogenesis

Transient monocular vision loss (TMVL), also referred to as **amaurosis fugax** ("fleeting blindness"), occurs from **retinal artery ischemia.** TMVL may result from vasospasm, flow lesions in the arterial supply to the retina, or emboli. Cholesterol emboli are most common and visualized funduscopically as Hollenhorst plaques. Thrombi may originate proximally (e.g., from the heart), embolizing through the internal carotid artery, to the ophthalmic artery, and finally to the retinal artery.

Epidemiology

Males are predominantly affected (2:1), especially white men. Risk factors for retinal ischemia include those commonly associated with **vascular disease:** hypertension, hypercholesterolemia, coronary artery disease, peripheral vascular disease, diabetes, male sex, smoking, and a positive family history.

Management

Stroke prevention. Carotid endarterectomy for symptomatic carotid artery stenosis of 70 to 99% is standard of care for prevention of stroke. **Aspirin** (pending no contraindications) in the perioperative period and indefinitely.

Complications

Persistent visual loss from retinal artery occlusion, stroke.

Breakout Point

- Amaurosis fugax results from retinal artery ischemia
- Associated with internal carotid artery stenosis

case 70

ID/CC	A **74-year-old African-American man** with a history of **hypertension** and **Type 2 diabetes mellitus** complains of sudden-onset **weakness in his right hand** and **drooling.**
HPI	He was asymptomatic when he went to bed, but when he woke up he noted clumsiness while brushing his teeth. He also noted drooling out of the right side of his mouth.
PE	VS: **hypertension** (BP 175/95). PE: alert and oriented; dysarthric; right facial droop with no forehead weakness (due to UMN right facial nerve palsy); motor strength 4/5 in right arm, 5/5 in right leg, and 5/5 in left arm and leg; reflexes 2+ and symmetric; Babinski's sign absent; sensory exam normal.
Labs	CBC: normal. Blood glucose elevated; **hypercholesterolemia** (LDL 295 mg/dL). ECG: sinus rhythm with LVH.
Imaging	CT brain (on admission): no mass; no shift; no hemorrhage; periventricular white matter disease consistent with small-vessel ischemia. CT head (24 hours after admission): lacunar ischemic infarct in the posterior limb of the left internal capsule (due to involvement of thalamoperforate arteries). US carotid: no significant stenosis. Echo: no thrombus; LVH.

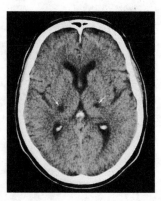

Figure 70-1. CT head: a different case showing bilateral lacunar infarcts.

139

case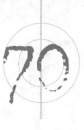

Stroke, Lacunar

Pathogenesis

Lacunar infarcts are caused by occlusion of penetrating branches of the circle of Willis, MCA, or vertebral and basilar arteries due to thrombosis or lipo-hyalinotic thickening of these branches.

Epidemiology

Lacunar strokes account for approximately 20% of all strokes.

Management

Antiplatelet agents (e.g., aspirin, ticlopidine) reduce stroke risk by 25%; begin after the initial head CT has ruled out cerebral hemorrhage. **Heparin** is given for DVT prophylaxis, and **lipid-lowering drugs** are given to reduce the risk of further strokes. Physical and occupational therapy are often useful in achieving maximal function.

Complications

Lacunar stroke patients have a 15% chance of recurrence after initial recovery, with an 8% mortality rate.

Breakout Point

- Lacunar infarcts are small lesions (<5 mm) in the basal ganglia, cerebellum, pons
- Associated with poorly controlled hypertension or diabetes

case 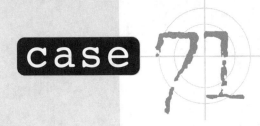 71

ID/CC An **82-year-old woman** with known dementia who resides at a nursing home presents with a change in mental status.

HPI The patient was in her usual state of health at dinner the previous night. In the morning, she complained of headache and could not move her right arm.

PE VS: no fever; **hypertension** (BP 160/95). PE: drowsy but able to follow simple commands; right facial droop noted; 0/5 strength in right arm and 4/5 strength in right leg; 5/5 strength in left arm and leg; DTRs 2+ in left arm and leg and **3+ in right arm and leg**; Babinski's sign absent.

Labs CBC/Lytes: normal. PT/PTT, glucose, BUN, and creatinine normal.

Imaging CT head: cortical hemorrhage in the left frontal lobe.

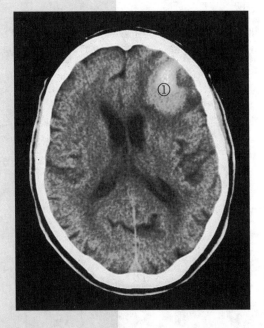

Figure 71-1. CT head: cortical hemorrhage in the left frontal lobe (1).

case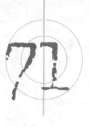

Stroke Due to Amyloid Angiopathy

Pathogenesis

Cerebral amyloid angiopathy (CAA) is characterized by **deposition of amyloid in small and medium-sized arteries in the cortex.** It has been associated with Alzheimer's disease but can also occur in otherwise healthy elderly patients. It may result in one or multiple simultaneous intracerebral, subarachnoid, or lobar hemorrhages. Clinical dementia is seen in 10 to 30% of patients with CAA. Pathologically, 50% present with neuritic plaques. The characteristic lesion is **Congo-red-positive, apple-green, birefringent** amyloid in the media and adventitia of arteries.

Epidemiology

Incidence increases with age; seen in 60% of autopsies in those older than 90 years.

Management

IV **beta-blockers** to keep systolic BP < 150.

Complications

Recurrent stroke.

Breakout Point

> Amyloid is Congo red positive and shows apple-green birefringence under polarized light.

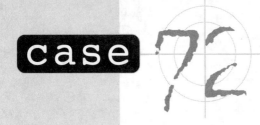
ID/CC	A **17-year-old boy** presents with **decreased level of consciousness.**
HPI	He was playing baseball when a friend accidentally hit him on the right side of the head with a bat. He **lost consciousness for less than 1 minute** but regained consciousness quickly with no obvious deficits, other than a **headache** over the right side of his head. He refused to go to the hospital. An hour later, he became **lethargic** and difficult to arouse and seemed **weak** on the **left** side of his body.
PE	VS: bradycardia and hypertensive (CUSHING REFLEX). PE: unconscious, making incomprehensible verbal responses. Eyes open only to pain. Pupils are unequal in size (ANISOCORIA); **right pupil is 6 mm with minimal reaction to light** (from compression of CN III). Right arm localizes to sternal rub, and right leg localizes pain. Left arm and leg extend to deep pain. **Babinski's sign** is present on the left. Glasgow Coma Scale: 9 (2+2+5).
Labs	CBC, BMP, LFTs, and coags are all normal.
Imaging	CT head: a lenticular (lens-shaped) hyperdense lesion in the right frontoparietal region.

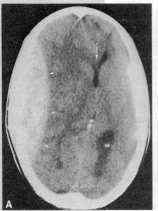
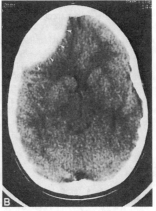

Figure 72-1. CT head (noncontrast): a lenticular (lens-shaped) hyperdense lesion (arrows) in the right frontoparietal region.

case 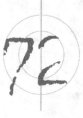 72

Epidural Hematoma

Pathogenesis

Epidural hematomas most commonly result from **lateral skull fractures** that **lacerate the middle meningeal artery.** Less than one-third of patients have a brief loss of consciousness followed by a **"lucid interval,"** where they regain consciousness, lasting minutes to hours and rarely 1 to 2 days, depending on the rate of blood accumulation between the dura and the skull. Gradual **progressive obtundation and hemiparesis** follow as the hematoma expands and compresses the temporal lobe, which may lead to transtentorial herniation. **Compression of CN III** results in a dilated and unreactive pupil suggestive of increased ICP or herniation. Compression of the cerebral peduncle causes contralateral weakness. Compression of the brain stem may also occur, causing ipsilateral weakness due to pyramidal tract dysfunction.

Epidemiology

Epidural hematoma constitutes 1 to 2% of all head trauma cases. A high mortality rate (up to 40%) is heralded by pupillary abnormalities, rapid clinical decline, temporal location, and age >55 or <5.

Management

Emergent surgical evacuation of the hematoma. Trephination (placement of a burr hole) may be necessary.

Complications

Death by herniation.

■ TABLE 72-1 GLASGOW COMA SCALE (GCS)

Category		Score
Eyes opening	Never	1
	To pain	2
	To verbal stimuli	3
	Spontaneously	4
Best verbal response	None	1
	Incomprehensible sounds	2
	Inappropriate words	3
	Disoriented and converses	4
	Oriented and converses	5
Best motor response	None	1
	Extension (decerebrate rigidity)	2
	Flexion (decorticate rigidity)	3
	Flexion withdrawal	4
	Patient localizes pain	5
	Patient obeys	6
TOTAL		3–15

Breakout Point

- Temporal skull fracture
- Middle meningeal artery laceration (arterial bleeding)
- Lens-shaped lesion on CT head
- Brief loss of consciousness followed by "lucid interval" before obtundation

case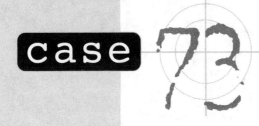

ID/CC A **57-year-old man** is brought to the emergency room by paramedics after a **motor vehicle accident.**

HPI A witness of the accident states that multiple cars were involved in the accident and that it took several hours for the patient to be extracted out of his car and brought to the hospital.

PE VS: **bradycardia** (HR 55) and **hypertensive** (BP 160/94) (Cushing reflex); tachypnea with stertorous breathing. PE: **somnolent** and responds only to deep, painful stimuli; left pupil is 7 mm and sluggishly reactive, while right pupil is 3 mm (left dilation indicating **uncal herniation**); patient demonstrates **decorticate posturing** (flexion of arms with extended legs); normal rectal tone; Babinski's sign (extensor plantar reflex) present on left; no other trauma present.

Labs CBC/Lytes: normal. Glucose, BUN/creatinine, and PT/PTT normal.

Imaging CT head: **hyperdense**, crescent-shaped **extra-axial fluid collection** showing mass effect (sulcal and ventricular effacement) and midline shift from left to right.

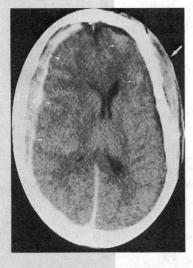

Figure 73-1. CT head: **hyperdense,** crescent-shaped **extra-axial fluid collection** showing mass effect (sulcal and ventricular effacement) and midline shift from left to right.

145

case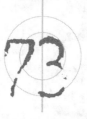

Subdural Hematoma—Acute

Pathogenesis

Subdural hematoma is an accumulation of blood between the **dura and arachnoid** due to disruption of the **bridging veins** that connect the cerebral cortex to the dural sinuses. The classic mechanism of injury is a **decelerating force** that tears veins. The hematoma displaces brain structures and may contribute to herniation; symptomatology may be minimal after trauma or may cause rapid death. Subdural hematomas may be divided into acute, subacute, and chronic forms. **Acute** subdural hematomas present in the first 24 hours after injury with a clinical picture of **severe neurologic damage**; bleeding is **venous** (in contrast to epidural hematomas). **Subacute** subdural hematomas present between 1 day and 2 weeks following injury; **progressive headache** is a common symptom, and there are usually focal neurologic signs. **Chronic subdural hematomas** are seen more frequently in **small infants and elderly** patients. They may follow trivial injuries to the head, are commonly bilateral, and occur 2 to 6 weeks after the injury; symptoms may include headache; balance difficulties or frequent falls; and confusion, seizures, or hemiparesis. MRI is better than CT for identifying a chronic subdural hematoma, as with chronicity the clot becomes isodense with brain tissue and may not be appreciated on a CT.

Epidemiology

The most common intracranial mass lesions resulting from trauma to the head. Patients with acute subdural hematoma have a **50% mortality rate.** The incidence of subdural hematoma increases with **age** (due to atrophy), **anticoagulant** use (mostly the subacute type), and **alcoholism** (due to frequent falls and atrophy).

Management

Intubate immediately and **hyperventilate** (to prevent cerebral vasodilation); load with **phenytoin** (to prevent **seizures**). Administer **mannitol** (to treat **cerebral edema**) and place the patient in **reverse Trendelenburg** position. **Surgical evacuation** of the hematoma is the mainstay of treatment.

Complications

Damage to the CNS may persist after surgical evacuation, increased ICP with herniation, and posttraumatic epilepsy.

Breakout Point

- Decelerating force
- Shearing of the bridging veins (venous bleeding)
- Crescentic (concave) hematomas on CT head
- Acute, subacute, chronic types

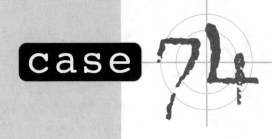

case 74

ID/CC A **52-year-old man** presents with **left eyelid droop** (PTOSIS) and **lack of perspiration** on the left side (ANHIDROSIS) following a motor vehicle accident.

HPI The patient has no significant medical history. His car was rear-ended at a traffic light.

PE VS: normal. PE: **left pupil constricted** (MIOSIS); left eyelid drooping; perspiration palpable on right side of forehead but not on left.

Labs CBC: normal. PT/PTT: normal.

Imaging US carotid: occlusion of the left internal carotid artery consistent with carotid dissection.

OTHER

case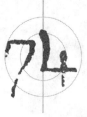

Horner's Syndrome

Pathogenesis

The course of the **sympathetic tract** can be disrupted at a number of sites, causing Horner's syndrome. The syndrome may be caused by any lesion that disrupts the sympathetic fibers in the carotid plexus, cervical sympathetic chain, upper thoracic cord (e.g., **superior sulcus or Pancoast's lung tumors**), or brain stem (**Wallenberg's syndrome**).

Epidemiology

The syndrome is relatively rare.

Management

Manage these patients in the **ICU**. When the cause of Horner's is carotid dissection, IV **heparin** and 3 to 6 months of **warfarin** is the accepted treatment. Prevention of unequal pupils is impossible. In cases in which trauma is not a potential cause, malignancy must be ruled out.

Breakout Point

- Ptosis, miosis, anhidrosis
- Due to disruption of the sympathetic tract

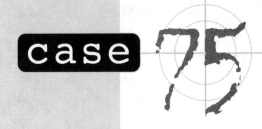

case 75

ID/CC	A **35-year-old man** complains of intermittent **episodes** of **nausea** and **dizziness** over the past month.
HPI	At first, the patient had episodes of nausea and a sensation that the **"room was spinning"** (VERTIGO); these episodes lasted 3 to 5 minutes. Over the past week, however, the symptoms have persisted for 1 to 2 hours. A severe episode 2 days ago resulted in emesis and "buzzing" in the left ear (TINNITUS).
PE	VS: normal. PE: mild sensorineural hearing loss in left ear; **Bárány maneuver** fails to reproduce sensation of vertigo; remainder of neurologic exam normal.
Labs	CBC: normal. Serum VDRL negative.
Imaging	MRI brain: unremarkable.

OTHER

case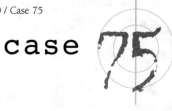

Ménière's Disease

Pathogenesis

Ménière's disease is caused by an **increase in volume of the endolymphatic system** (ENDOLYMPHATIC HYDROPS), resulting in distention. The primary lesion is thought to be in the endolymphatic sac, which is responsible for endolymph filtration and excretion. Two known causes are syphilis and head trauma.

Epidemiology

Typical onset is in middle age.

Management

Treat acute attacks with **bed rest; meclizine** or **dimenhydrinate** is used for symptomatic relief of vertigo. Chronic treatment involves institution of a **low-sodium diet** and **diuretics**. To treat intractable disease, a **surgical shunt** should be placed (relieves vertigo in 70% of cases but causes hearing loss in 50%).

Complications

Remissions and relapses may occur throughout life; gradual **hearing loss** due to multiple attacks is possible.

Breakout Point

> • Vertigo, tinnitus, hearing loss, feeling of fullness, or blockage in ear

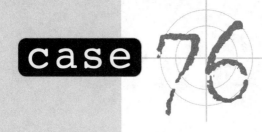

case 76

ID/CC	A **25-year-old white woman** presents to her primary care doctor for **excessive daytime sleepiness** that started about 10 years ago.
HPI	She states, "I can't seem to stay awake in the day." She also describes episodes of **paralysis** on awakening (SLEEP PARALYSIS) and **dream-like hallucinations** as she falls asleep (HYPNAGOGIC HALLUCINATIONS). When laughing at a joke or angry, she sometimes feels **weak in her knees** and almost collapses to the floor (CATA-PLEXY). These episodes occur about once a month. She describes herself as a "sleepy person" and feels **refreshed by short naps**.
PE	VS: normal. Height and weight normal for age. HEENT: no signs of obstruction (sleep apnea less likely); neurologic exam normal.
Labs	CBC/Lytes: normal. **HLA-DR2** testing was positive.
Imaging	None.

OTHER

151

case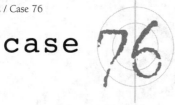

Narcolepsy

Pathogenesis

Narcolepsy is an often unrecognized disorder that is thought to be related to a genetic abnormality, neuropeptide deficiency (hypocretin), and abnormal immune system regulation. There is disruption of the "sleep–wake" cycle specifically with REM sleep and defects in the pontine reticular activating system. Narcolepsy with cataplexy is strongly associated with **HLA-DR2** (in Caucasian patients) and **HLA DQB1* 0602** in other ethnic groups.

Epidemiology

Incidence is comparable to multiple sclerosis. Bimodal distribution of age-of-onset: 15 (highest peak) and 36.

Management

Overnight sleep study (**polysomnogram**) to rule out sleep apnea followed by a mean sleep latency test (**MSLT**), which is four or five 20-minute nap trials to measure REM latency. Sleep hygiene: adequate sleep and planned naps. Improve wakefulness with **stimulants** (e.g., methylphenidate) or stimulant-like medications (e.g., modafinil). Treat cataplexy with tricyclic antidepressants or SSRIs.

Complications

Low sex drive or even impotence. **Sleep attacks** can lead to serious injury, e.g., while driving.

Breakout Point

> Tetrad of Narcolepsy:
> - Excessive daytime sleepiness
> - Cataplexy (abrupt attack of muscle weakness triggered by emotion)
> - Hypnagogic hallucinations
> - Paralysis on waking

questions

1. A previously healthy 30-year-old woman presents with intermittent attacks of intense vertigo for the past 2 months. Each attack lasts for a few hours and is accompanied by nausea, tinnitus, and a feeling of fullness in her left ear. Physical examination reveals mild nystagmus, which is most exaggerated with gaze to the right. Cranial nerve testing is normal. Ocular examination shows no palsies. Romberg and heel-to-toe walking is within normal limits. Audiogram testing demonstrates decreased high-pitched tone hearing in her left ear. Which of the following is the most likely diagnosis?

   A. Otitis media
   B. Labyrinthitis
   C. Acoustic neuroma
   D. Multiple sclerosis
   E. Ménière's disease

2. A 40-year-old man presents with numbness and tingling in his arms for the past day. Following a car accident 2 days ago, he was assessed in the emergency room, and was found to have a normal neurologic examination. He reports aching in both shoulders and arms. Numbness and tingling is exacerbated by reaching up for items on high shelves, and symptoms are relieved by rest. He has not used acetaminophen or NSAIDs for pain relief. Current neurologic examination reveals decreased pinprick sensation and weakness in the first three digits on both hands and weakness of shoulder abduction bilaterally. Biceps reflex is diminished on the left side. Which of the following is the next step in management?

   A. MRI of neck
   B. Surgical decompression
   C. Soft cervical collar
   D. Epidural corticosteroids
   E. Morphine

3. A 25-year-old man is found unconscious in a parking lot near his car. He was unaccompanied and the state surrounding this incident was not witnessed. Physical examination shows that he is breathing normally, with good capillary refill and pink mucous membranes. A small bleeding laceration is noted on the right side of his head. Which of the following factors is the most specific in indicating that he had a seizure before he lost consciousness?

A. Bite marks on his tongue
B. Brief tonic-clonic movements before falling
C. Confusion and sleepiness on awakening
D. Sensation of palpitations before falling
E. An aura of nausea before falling

4. A 40-year-old woman presents with complaints of fasciculations and discomfort in both legs that has progressed over the past week. She also has nonradiating pain in her lower back that is worse when she bends down to pick up her young son. She denies urinary or bowel incontinence, numbness, tingling, or change in sensation. Neurologic examination shows normal strength, normal sensation to light touch and pinprick, and normal patellar and Achilles reflex bilaterally. Leg raise is negative bilaterally, but pain is elicited with palpation over the lumbar spine. Which of the following is the next step in management?

A. MRI of spine
B. CT of spine
C. Electromyography (EMG)
D. Ultrasound of the lower extremities
E. Reassurance

5. A 62-year-old man presents with progressive weakness in his legs over the past 2 weeks. He reports mild electric shock-like pain shooting down his buttocks and the backs of his legs. He denies history of trauma, excessive exertion, fever, or intravenous drug use. Physical examination reveals bilateral lower extremity weakness which is more pronounced on the right side, decreased sensation in a band-like region at T11 that descends to both lower extremities, and spasticity and clonus on reflex testing. Which of the following is the most likely diagnosis?

A. Glioblastoma multiforme
B. Ependymoma
C. Astrocytoma
D. Primary CNS lymphoma
E. Medulloblastoma

6. A 52-year-old woman presents with a fractured right wrist after a fall. She complains of unsteadiness and difficulty walking for the past four months. She reports burning "prickly" pain in her feet when she tries to sleep at night. She has difficulty in balancing herself when she stands up from a sitting position. Physical examination demonstrates swaying when she stands from a chair. She falls over when she attempts to stand with her feet together, with her eyes open or closed. Gait is unstable with a wide-based stance. Sensory loss is noted in her feet. Which of the following is the most likely diagnosis?

A. Subacute combined degeneration of the spinal cord
B. Neurosyphilis
C. Normal pressure hydrocephalus
D. Alcoholic cerebellar degeneration
E. Parkinson disease

7. A 59-year-old right-handed man presents to an outpatient clinic with an intermittent tremor in his right hand and complains of a stiff and aching right arm for the past several weeks. His temperature was 98.4°F, blood pressure 140/80 mm Hg, pulse 96/min, respirations 18/min, and oxygen saturation 98% on room air. Physical examination shows a mild rest tremor in the right hand that disappears when he writes his name and moderate rigidity at the right wrist and elbow. Finger tapping is slowed in the right. He walks slowly with a short-stepped gait and has a decreased arm swing on the right. His right hand tremor is more notable when he walks. He is bothered by these symptoms and wants to be treated. Which of the following interventions would be most appropriate?

    A. CT of head
    B. Amantadine
    C. Risperidone
    D. Physostigmine
    E. No pharmacologic intervention

Questions 8 and 9

A 21-year-old woman presents with blurry vision in her right eye that has been progressing for the past four days. Before this change in her vision, she complained of a dull ache behind her right eye that worsened with eye movement. She has no past history of visual or neurological problems. Physical exam reveals visual acuity of 20/60 in the right eye with a central visual field loss. Color perception is reduced; specifically, the color red appeared "washed out." A right afferent pupillary defect was demonstrated by a swinging flashlight test, where the right pupil responded poorly to light stimulation compared with the left pupil. On funduscopic exam, there is visible swelling of the optic disk. A comprehensive neurological examination is normal. CBC, BMP, and ESR are all normal.

8. Based on these symptoms, which of following diseases would be most necessary to evaluate?

    A. Multiple sclerosis
    B. Cluster headache
    C. Transient monocular vision loss (amaurosis fugax)
    D. Temporal arteritis
    E. Acute angle-closure glaucoma

9. How would this condition be best evaluated further?

   A. Biopsy of temporal artery
   B. Lumbar puncture
   C. CT of head and spine
   D. MRI of brain and spine
   E. Carotid artery doppler

10. A 35-year-old man with no medical problems notices that the left side of his face is drooping one day before visiting the emergency room. On physical examination, there is obvious facial asymmetry. When asked to close his eyes tightly, his left eye remains partially open; however, he is able to move both eyes in all directions. When asked to smile, he cannot show you his teeth; also, he cannot inflate his cheek on the left. What medical treatment can be offered to treat the condition that is most likely responsible for his symptoms?

    A. Oral prednisone and acyclovir
    B. IV heparin and warfarin
    C. Aspirin
    D. IM ceftriaxone
    E. Lumbar puncture

11. A previously healthy 12-year-old boy is brought to his pediatrician by his mother. He woke up this morning and found that he could not move the left side of his face. He denies fevers, visual changes, rashes, or trauma. For the past several days, he complained to his mother he was having pain in both of his knees, and he recovered from the "flu" about 6 weeks ago after they went on a hiking trip; his mom noted that he had a rash on his leg at the time. Physical exam reveals an afebrile boy with knees with bilateral effusions and pain with motion. He has a left facial droop of both the upper and lower face. The rest of the physical exam is unremarkable. What is the most likely diagnosis?

    A. Ramsay Hunt syndrome
    B. Lyme disease
    C. Right-sided stroke
    D. Myasthenia gravis
    E. Multiple sclerosis

12. A 49-year-old man with no known chronic medical illness has an episode of weakness of his left face, arm, and leg accompanied by difficulty speaking. By the time he arrives in the ED (30 minutes after the onset of his symptoms), he is noted to have full strength of all extremities and no dysarthria. His heart rhythm is noted to be irregularly irregular with a pulse in the 120s. A head CT is negative for

infarct, bleed, or mass. Doppler ultrasonography of the carotid arteries is negative for thrombus or atherosclerotic plaque. Which of the following is the most appropriate treatment?

A. Initiate aspirin and discharge for outpatient follow-up.
B. Admit the patient to control the rate of his pulse with a calcium-channel blocker, begin aspirin, and anticoagulate with heparin.
C. Admit the patient to control the rate of his pulse with a calcium-channel blocker.
D. Attempt vagal maneuvers to convert rhythm and initiate aspirin and anticoagulation with heparin.
E. Initiate aspirin and calcium-channel blocker and discharge for outpatient follow-up.

13. A 34-year-old man was admitted for laparoscopic cholecystectomy. He is otherwise well and takes no medications. Postoperatively, he complained of mild to moderate pain and was given Tylenol with codeine for pain control. He also has nausea and vomiting and is unable to keep any fluids down. Metoclopramide (Reglan™) is given intravenously for nausea. After the second dose, he calls the nurses because of pain in his eyes. On examination, his eyes are deviated upward and slightly to the right. His neck is stiff and held in slight extension and lateral flexion to the right. His mental status is intact and the rest of the neurological examination is normal. The most appropriate treatment of his condition is:

A. Haldol
B. Aspirin
C. Ceftriaxone
D. Phenytoin
E. Benztropine

14. A 55-year-old man was admitted to the hospital after he sustained a hip fracture from falling down a flight of stairs. He was immediately taken to the operating room for open reduction internal fixation and did well after the surgery. On hospital day 3, he said that there were people in his room (when there were none) and began crying out at them. He also became very agitated and tried to climb out of the bed. He had a fever of 100.6°F, blood pressure 180/90 mm Hg, pulse 140/min, respirations 22/min, and oxygen saturation 98% on room air. He was diaphoretic and tremulous. He was very inattentive and would not cooperate with the full mental status examination. There were no localizing features on his neurologic examination. His wife states that he typically drinks "a couple of glasses of wine" with dinner everyday. The most appropriate treatment for his condition is:

A. Haldol
B. Acyclovir
C. Lorazepam
D. Propranolol
E. Phenytoin

15. A 52-year-old African-American man with a history of tobacco use and poorly controlled hypertension was carrying groceries home one day, when suddenly he had a severe right-sided headache, followed by left-sided numbness and weakness. He was brought to the emergency room, where his temperature was 98.6°F, blood pressure 186/100 mm Hg, pulse 96/min, respirations 14/min, and oxygen saturation 98% on room air. Physical examination shows a left facial droop with significant weakness of the left lower half of the face, slightly dysphasic speech, and left arm and leg weakness. He also has diminished sensation to pain, temperature, vibration, and joint position sense in the left arm and leg. There is also diminished sensation to the pain and temperature on the left side of his trunk. A noncontrast CT of the head shows a hyperdense lesion in the right thalamus and internal capsular region, consistent with an acute hemorrhage. The most likely etiology of his intracerebral hemorrhage is:

A. Arteriovenous malformation
B. Amyloid angiopathy
C. Metastatic lesion
D. Hypertension
E. Cerebral aneurysm

16. A 22-year-old woman comes into the office complaining of recurrent episodes of visual disturbances. She describes flashing lights, zigzag lines in the central portion of her visual field, which last 20 minutes and then resolve spontaneously. This is then followed by a severe pounding headache in the right frontal region, associated with nausea, vomiting, photophobia and phonophobia, unrelieved by ibuprofen or acetaminophen. When she goes to take a nap in a dark quiet room, she feels much better. She is otherwise healthy. Both her mother and her older sister have similar conditions. Neurologic examination is normal. The most effective medication for treating the acute symptoms of her condition is:

A. Phenytoin
B. Acetaminophen
C. Propranolol
D. Sumatriptan
E. Risperidone

17. A 16-year-old girl with no significant past medical history was brought to the emergency room by her parents because of headache, neck stiffness, and fever since this morning. Over the past several hours, she has become very sleepy. On examination, she is febrile with a temperature of 102°F, blood pressure 110/70 mm Hg, pulse 98/min, respirations 16/min, and oxygen saturation 98% on room air. She is lethargic and needs constant stimulation to remain awake. She has nuchal rigidity and Kernig's sign is present. She also has a petechial rash on her body and limbs. The most appropriate next step in management is:

    A. Head CT
    B. Lumbar puncture
    C. EEG
    D. Initiate broad spectrum antibiotics
    E. Obtain blood cultures

18. A 32-year-old woman presents to the emergency room with double vision. She had a mild cough and rhinorrhea several days ago because of a cold that is currently resolving. She has also been feeling fatigued in the evening and has trouble climbing up the stairs to her bedroom. She initially attributed her symptoms to the cold, but became alarmed when she noticed intermittent double vision for the past 2 days. She is typically fine in the morning, but by the end of the day, she has significant intermittent double vision, particularly on looking to the right. On examination, her pupils are normal but she has mild bilateral ptosis and which becomes much more pronounced after sustained upgaze for 60 seconds. On lateral gaze, there is limited adduction in both eyes, but more prominent in the left eye. There is mild weakness of neck flexion and shoulder abduction. Her sensory exam and reflexes are intact. The most appropriate diagnostic test to perform next is:

    A. MRI of the brain
    B. Lumbar puncture
    C. Edrophonium test
    D. Nerve conduction study
    E. Muscle biopsy

19. A 56-year-old man presents to the emergency room because of facial droop. Two days ago, he had pain in the right ear. Since yesterday, he has had progressive right facial droop. His coworkers noticed an asymmetric smile and his face seems to be pulled to the left side. He is also unable to close the right eye completely and noticed increased tearing in the right eye. When he is waiting for the train in the subway, the loud noise created by the trains produces significant discomfort in the right ear. On examination, he has flat right nasolabial fold.

He is unable to raise his right eyebrow and when he tries to close the right eye, the eyeball deviates upward (Bell's phenomenon). He also has weakness on the right side when he smiles and is unable to whistle. Taste is absent over the anterior portion the tongue on the right to sugar and salt. Examination of the ears reveals vesicular eruptions in the internal auditory canal on the right. The most likely etiology of his symptoms is:

A. Lyme disease
B. Ramsey Hunt syndrome
C. Sarcoidosis
D. Ischemic Stroke
E. Tumor

20. A 50-year-old woman with a history of hypertension and hypercholesterolemia presents to the emergency room with two episodes of visual disturbance in the left eye while she was reading her music during choir practice. It was as if there was a curtain descending over her left eye for a couple of minutes. During one of the episodes, she tried to test her vision by closing either eye and noticed that the vision was completely normal in the right eye. She denied any pain in the eyes and reported no sensory disturbances or weakness during the episodes. On physical examination, she has a bruit over the left anterior neck region. Her neurological examination is normal. The most likely etiology of her symptom is:

A. Migraine
B. Partial seizure
C. Acute angle closure glaucoma
D. Optic neuritis
E. Amaurosis fugax

answers

1-E

A. Otitis media [Incorrect] typically presents as pain in the inner ear, fever, and muffled hearing, but vertigo is unusual. Otitis media is usually preceded or intercurrent with an upper respiratory tract infection.

B. Labyrinthitis [Incorrect] is an inflammation of the vestibular labyrinth (canals and cavities in the inner ear). In contrast to Ménière's disease, patients with labyrinthitis have acute episodes of vertigo (lasting <1 minute) associated with turning of the head or head movement. Hearing loss and repeated episodes over months is rare.

C. Acoustic neuroma [Incorrect] rarely causes vertigo, and any associated vertigo is usually mild.

D. Multiple sclerosis [Incorrect] is an autoimmune demyelinating disease of the CNS. Initial presentation is classically optic neuritis, decrease in fine motor coordination, or myelitis, with brainstem signs.

E. Ménière's disease [Correct] is characterized by attacks of vertigo, nausea, vomiting, tinnitus, high-pitched tone hearing loss, and a feeling of fullness in the ear.

2-C

A. MRI of neck [Incorrect] would not be performed at this time. Although the imaging method of choice in cervical radiculopathy, incidental abnormalities have been noted in asymptomatic patients, making interpretation of findings difficult. Imaging is performed in the context of the severity and duration of examination findings.

B. Surgical decompression [Incorrect] is too aggressive at this time. The goal of management is to reduce inflammation with rest and medications as an outpatient, to determine if symptoms will resolve without invasive therapy.

C. This patient has cervical radiculopathy from herniation of a lower cervical disk. His symptoms were likely precipitated from preceding trauma and possible neck hyperextension during the car accident. Cervical radiculopathy is managed conservatively as an outpatient, with soft cervical collar [Correct], ice, rest, and NSAIDs to reduce inflammation.

D. Epidural corticosteroids [Incorrect] are also too aggressive at this time. NSAIDs should be initiated first.

E. Morphine [Incorrect] would not be as effective as NSAIDs in decreasing inflammation, and it is not part of first-line treatment.

3-C

A. Although biting of the tongue [Incorrect] can occur during a seizure, it is not pathognomic for seizure and also can occur during syncope and from fall trauma.

B. Brief tonic-clonic movements before falling [Incorrect] can also be witnessed in other clinical states, such as hypoglycemia, infection, electrolyte disturbances, or brain tumor.

C. A patient who has a seizure that induces loss of consciousness will typically demonstrate a postictal state of confusion, sleepiness, lack of awareness on awakening [Correct]. Neurologic deficits such as Todd's paralysis can occur in a postictal state. Immediate alertness on awakening should provoke suspicion for an alternative diagnosis.

D. A sensation of palpitations before falling [Incorrect] is the most common cardiac manifestation to precede a seizure, but isolated arrhythmias without seizure can also induce loss of consciousness.

E. An aura of nausea before falling [Incorrect] can occur before a seizure, but nausea is a nonspecific symptom that does not necessarily indicate that a seizure has occurred.

4-E

A. MRI of spine [Incorrect] should be performed in the context of a concurrent diagnosis such as cancer (possible metastases), an abnormal neurologic exam, or with reports of urinary or bowel incontinence, inability to move one or both legs, or loss of sensation in the legs. Isolated fasciculations, discomfort, and mild lower back pain are not indications for imaging.

B. If imaging is indicated, CT of spine [Incorrect] would not be the imaging modality of choice, since a concerning history and physical requires assessment with MRI of spine.

C. In electromyography (EMG) [Incorrect], a thin needle electrode is inserted into muscle, and the size, duration, and frequency of electrical signals are compared at rest and with activity. Nerve conduction studies are also performed. EMG is used to diagnose diseases such as muscular dystrophy, peripheral neuropathies, and myasthenia gravis, among others, but would not be indicated for this patient's symptoms.

D. Ultrasound of the lower extremities [Incorrect] is performed when there is high suspicion for deep vein thromboses, the presence of which manifests as discomfort and asymmetric swelling of the legs.

E. Fasciculations and discomfort in the legs can be noted in conditions such as amyotrophic lateral sclerosis, ruptured intervertebral disk, electrolyte abnormalities, toxin ingestion, or excessive caffeine ingestion. In the absence of neurologic findings, patients should be given reassurance [Correct] and managed conservatively on an outpatient basis.

5-B

A. Glioblastoma multiforme [Incorrect] is the most common and the most malignant of glial tumors, but it most commonly occurs in the cerebral hemispheres. It is very rarely found in the spine.

B. Ependymomas [Correct] are glial tumors that arise from ependymal cells of the CNS. In adults, the majority of ependymomas occur in the spinal canal, which can cause neurologic deficits characteristic of a root level lesion.

C. Astrocytomas [Incorrect] are CNS tumors of astrocytes. They can arise at any site in the CNS, but astrocytomas of the spinal cord are uncommon.

D. Primary CNS lymphoma [Incorrect] is a rare high-grade, non-Hodgkin B cell neoplasm, most commonly a diffuse large B cell lymphoma. It most commonly occurs in the context of immunosuppression, and is thus suspected in patients with AIDS or transplant patients.

E. Medulloblastoma [Incorrect] is a primitive neuroectodermal tumor (PNET) that most commonly arises in the posterior fossa. It can occur at any age, but is predominantly a pediatric tumor that arises in the cerebellum.

6-D

A. Subacute combined degeneration of the spinal cord [Incorrect] refers to neuropathy that develops in the context of vitamin B_{12} deficiency, affecting the posterior and lateral columns of the spinal cord. The classic triad is numbness/paresthesias, weakness, and a sore, red beefy tongue. Because liver stores are high (2 to 4 mg), vitamin B_{12} deficiency occurs over years to decades.

B. Neurosyphilis [Incorrect] is a sign of tertiary syphilis, which manifests with cognitive deficits, personality changes, or psychiatric disturbance. It is preceded by infection with *Treponema pallidum*, the causative organism of syphilis.

C. Normal pressure hydrocephalus [Incorrect] manifests as the classic triad of dementia, urinary incontinence, and gait instability (mnemonic: "wacky, water, walking"). Radiologic imaging of the head demonstrates ventricular dilation, with a normal CSF opening pressure on lumbar puncture.

D. Alcoholic cerebellar degeneration [Correct] primarily affects the midline cerebellar vermis, classically the superior portion more than the inferior portion. This condition is associated with a history of long-term alcohol abuse, and a slow chronic process of motor, sensory, and wide-based gait disturbance that develops over months.

E. Parkinson disease [Incorrect] is a neurodegenerative disease attributed to loss of dopaminergic neurons in the substantia nigra. Characteristic signs include an asymmetric resting tremor, bradykinesia, rigidity, and a shuffling gait.

7-B

A. Head CT [Incorrect] is not a primary diagnostic tool for the evaluation of Parkinson's disease, which can be diagnosed clinically. MR imaging of the brain may be useful in a patient with prominent gait abnormalities to exclude other conditions, but the diagnosis of Parkinson's disease can be made by careful history and physical examination.

B. Amantadine [Correct] is an NMDA antagonist used as an adjunctive agent to treat Parkinson's disease. Amantadine has fewer adverse effects but only moderate effect in treating symptoms. It generally needs to be combined with another agent, like levodopa, to adequately treat symptoms.

C. Risperidone [Incorrect] is an atypical antipsychotic with prominent D2 blockade. Parkinsonism is often induced by antipsychotic medications, and risperidone is a common culprit. Initiation of risperidone would worsen this patient's symptoms and is not indicated.

D. Physostigmine [Incorrect] is a reversible cholinesterase inhibitor that crosses the blood-brain barrier and would increase the available amount of acetylcholine at the postsynaptic neuromuscular junction. Parkinson's disease can be treated with anticholinergics, not cholinomimetics, so this intervention would be contraindicated. Anticholinergic agents, like benztropine, are sometimes added to treat a tremor refractory to other medications, but they generally are not used because of adverse effects.

E. Although his symptoms are mild overall, this patient is sufficiently bothered by the symptoms to request treatment for them. He may respond well to a trial of the most effective agent, levodopa, and amantadine may be initiated with this dopamine precursor or at a later time. Withholding treatment (no pharmacological intervention) would not be the best approach [Incorrect].

8-A

A. This patient has a classic presentation for optic neuritis. The most common form of optic neuritis is acute demyelinating optic neuritis, which is highly associated with multiple sclerosis [Correct], occurring in half of cases and often as the presenting complaint. The presence of an afferent pupillary defect is correlative to optic neuritis. Absence of this finding in patients with acute visual loss suggests retinal disease or bilateral optic-nerve dysfunction. This patient also has a central scotoma, a classic finding in optic neuritis. The presence of papillitis (swelling of the optic disk) is only present in one-third of cases; most cases have normal optic disks, described as retrobulbar optic neuritis.

B. Cluster headache [Incorrect] often presents in patients in their 20s and with orbital pain, but this patient did not have an acute onset of symptoms, which would be more suggestive of cluster headache. The presence of an afferent pupillary defect suggests a more discrete diagnosis.

C. Amaurosis fugax [Incorrect] typically occurs in older patients with risk factors for stroke. Vision loss associated with amaurosis fugax is fleeting (not progressive, as was noted in this patient) and is often described as a shade being pulled down (not as a central scotoma).

D. Temporal arteritis [Incorrect] is an important alternate diagnosis, but it occurs more often in the elderly and would be associated with a highly elevated ESR.

E. By history, there are several features in this case that would indicate acute angle-closure glaucoma [Incorrect], including blurry vision, periorbital pain, visual deficits, and ipsilateral headache. However, the onset of symptoms, as the name of the diagnosis indicates, is acute and severe, and patients are typically elderly and hyperopic (farsighted).

9-D

A. Biopsy of temporal artery [Incorrect] would be too invasive a diagnostic procedure in a patient of this age with a normal ESR and no scalp tenderness, with a diagnosis better explained by optic neuritis.

B. Lumbar puncture [Incorrect] in a patient with multiple sclerosis would reveal oligoclonal banding of proteins; in a patient without a previous diagnosis of multiple sclerosis, presence of this marker may predict development of multiple sclerosis. This would also be a useful diagnostic intervention for this patient, but MRI would be a better choice if only one intervention can be chosen.

C. CT of head and spine [Incorrect] would not allow for adequate visualization of plaques in the white matter as compared to MRI.

D. Acute demyelinating optic neuritis can be diagnosed clinically, but because of the high association with multiple sclerosis, evaluation for demyelinating lesions with MRI is necessary. Risk for development of multiple sclerosis is best evaluated with gadolinium-enhanced MRI of the brain [Correct] to identify any suggestive white-matter lesions, which would be treated with intravenous methylprednisolone followed by oral prednisone taper. Treatment with interferon beta-1a or interferon beta-1b also may be considered.

E. Doppler of carotid arteries (Incorrect) would be appropriate to evaluate atherosclerotic plaques in a patient with risk factors or clinical signs and symptoms suggestive of stroke or transient monocular vision loss. This patient's vision changes are better explained by optic neuritis.

10-A

A. Oral prednisone and acyclovir [Correct]. This patient presents with symptoms that are highly suggestive of Bell's palsy. Evaluation of this patient begins by determining if the lesion is central or peripheral. Involvement of both the upper and lower face without an apparent cause increases the likelihood of Bell's palsy. No tests are indicated if there are no other cranial nerve deficits, and a diagnosis is made within 1 week of symptoms, as in this case. According to the Quality Standards Subcommittee of the American Academy of Neurology, early treatment with oral corticosteroids [Correct] is probably effective in improving facial-function outcomes in Bell's palsy (and decreasing the incidence of permanent facial paralysis). HSV-1 DNA appears to be specific to Bell's palsy; it does not correlate with Ramsay Hunt syndrome or other neurologic diseases. Also, the addition of acyclovir to prednisone is possibly effective. Insufficient evidence exists to recommend facial-nerve decompression.

B. IV heparin and warfarin [Incorrect] would be a treatment of choice in a patient with atrial fibrillation who suffers a stroke, but there is no history given of atrial fibrillation in this patient, and his lesion appears to be peripheral.

C. Initiating aspirin [Incorrect] would be appropriate for a patient who presents with symptoms of stroke, but this patient's symptoms are better explained by a peripheral lesion.

D. IM ceftriaxone [Incorrect] would be an appropriate treatment for bacterial meningitis, but this patient does not have any of the cardinal features of this illness.

E. Lumbar puncture [Incorrect] would be therapeutic in a patient with idiopathic intracranial hypertension; this may present with subacute headache, vomiting, and blurred vision, as well as visual disturbance with postural change, particularly in an obese woman.

11-B

A. Ramsay Hunt syndrome [Incorrect] often presents with unilateral facial weakness, hearing loss, and ear pain that is associated with vesicular herpes zoster infection. Although this boy has unilateral facial weakness, the constellation of symptoms associated with Ramsay Hunt is lacking.

B. This boy is in the second stage of Lyme disease [Correct], a tick-borne, spirochetal illness resulting from infection with *Borrelia burgdorferi*. It presents in three clinical stages. The first stage includes flu-like symptoms, and 50% of patients have the classic rash of erythema chronicum migrans, an expanding erythematous area with central clearing. This patient likely contracted Lyme disease from a tick while on a hiking trip and developed flu-like symptoms and a rash shortly thereafter. The second stage, which occurs weeks to months later, can include arthritis of the large joints and neurological symptoms; in this case, he developed a Bell's palsy. Cardiac symptoms, including heart block, can also be seen in the second stage.

C. A right-sided stroke [Incorrect] would be unlikely in a young boy with no history of coagulopathy or disease predisposing to labile blood pressure. Also, the presence of an upper motor neuron lesion, unless the facial nucleus were involved, would lead to facial weakness in the lower face alone. Lesions of cranial nerve VII, or Bell's palsy, are commonly seen in Lyme disease.

D. Myasthenia gravis [Incorrect] is a disease of the neuromuscular junction that can cause bilateral (not unilateral) facial weakness as well as weakness in other muscles. Weakness is often most notable in the extraocular and eyelid muscles. Affiliated symptoms of a rash and inflammatory arthritis of the knees would not be indicative of an episode of myasthenia gravis.

E. Although multiple sclerosis [Incorrect] can have highly variable presentations, including neurological weakness, the presence of a single episode would not allow for a diagnosis of MS, which necessitates multiple episodes separated in time (and lesions occurring in different spaces).

12-B

A. To initiate aspirin and discharge to outpatient follow-up [Incorrect] might be appropriate in a patient who reports symptoms of a TIA that last less than 10 minutes with a negative head CT, normal carotid Doppler, unremarkable labs, and low risk factors for stroke. This patient has a new onset atrial fibrillation that likely produced an embolus causing TIA that needs rate control and anticoagulation to prevent a stroke.

B. The use of heparin [Correct] in patients with brain hemorrhage is usually not justified, but in this patient it would be appropriate to reduce the high short-term risk of stroke following a TIA in a patient with atrial fibrillation. This patient has had a transient ischemic attack. A commonly accepted definition of TIA is based on clinical findings as a neurologic deficit lasting less than 24 hours that is attributed to focal cerebral or retinal ischemia. Common risk factors include those that predispose to stroke, e.g., atrial fibrillation, carotid-artery disease, and large- and small-artery disease in the brain. This patient presented with a new-onset atrial fibrillation. If the short-term risk for stroke is high, then urgent evaluation and treatment following TIA is necessary. Risk factors that may predispose to stroke in patients with TIA include advanced age, diabetes, duration of symptoms for more than 10 minutes, and weakness or speech impairment with the episode. Although evaluation within the first day is required, hospitalization is indicated only if the evaluation cannot be completed.

In most patients, aspirin will be the initial treatment of choice (clopidogrel and aspirin + dipyridamole are alternatives). Atrial fibrillation needs to be rate controlled (often with a beta blocker or calcium-channel blocker), and anticoagulation can begin with a plan to transition heparin (either unfractionated or low molecular weight) to warfarin.

C. While admitting the patient and starting a calcium-channel blocker [Incorrect] are both appropriate interventions, this answer does not fully address the risk for further emboli.

D. Vagal maneuvers [Incorrect] would be appropriate for a patient with a supraventricular tachycardia, which may convert the rhythm to normal sinus rhythm. These maneuvers would include carotid massage or bearing down. This patient's irregularly irregular rhythm is more indicative of atrial fibrillation.

E. Though starting aspirin and a calcium-channel blocker are correct interventions [Incorrect], the patient would require further inpatient monitoring to ensure that the rate of the rhythm remains controlled over time. This choice also does not address the need for initiating anticoagulation, which would also require an inpatient hospitalization in this setting.

13-E

A. Haldol [Incorrect] is a typical neuroleptic with significant D2 receptor blocking activity and would exacerbate the condition.

B. These symptoms are not likely due to acute stroke given the temporal relationship with metochlopramide use. Thus, aspirin [Incorrect] would not be appropriate.

C. Ceftriaxone [Incorrect] is not appropriate as this is not due to infection.

D. Phenytoin [Incorrect] is also not appropriate as his ocular and torticollis are not due to seizures.

E. This man has the classic symptoms of oculogyric crisis and torticollis, a form of dystonic reaction, as a complication of metoclopramide. Acute dystonic reactions are extrapyramidal side effects to medications that block the D2 receptor, such as neuroleptics and antiemetics such as metoclopramide or prochloperazine. Men and younger patients are at higher risk and symptoms may occur within 1 week of drug administration, although the typical time period is within 48 hours. The treatment of choice is intravenous anticholinergic agents such as benztropine [Correct] or diphenhydramine.

14-C

A. Haldol [Incorrect] may be administered for hallucinations or aggressive behavior, but it is not the treatment of choice for delirium tremens.

B. Viral encephalitis with herpes simplex is unlikely in this case given the constellation of the clinical syndrome and the temporal relationship with cessation of alcohol. Thus, acyclovir [Incorrect] would not be an appropriate choice of treatment.

C. This man is most likely suffering from delirium tremens, a potentially fatal form of alcohol withdrawal which typically manifests 48 to 72 hours after the last drink. Although his wife states that he drinks only "a couple of glasses of wine" every night, this is likely an underestimate of his true alcohol consumption. The proposed mechanism is upregulation of glutamate receptors and downregulation of GABA receptors. The mortality is up to 15% for delirium tremens if untreated. Clinically, it is typically characterized by delirium, hallucinations (visual, auditory, tactile), agitation, and tremor. Autonomic instability (including fever, diaphoresis, tachycardia, hypertension, and tachypnea) is a hallmark of the condition. Treatment of delirium tremens involves benzodiazepines such as lorazepam [Correct], which can be tapered after 1 to 2 days.

D. Propranolol [Incorrect] may be appropriate for patients who demonstrate hypertension and tachycardia due to sudden withdrawal of chronic beta blockage. However, patients do not typically have delirium or hallucinations.

E. Phenytoin [Incorrect] is typically not effective in preventing alcohol withdrawal seizures.

15-D

A. Arteriovenous malformations [Incorrect] are congenital abnormal connections between the arterial and venous bed, where a mature capillary bed fails to form. These malformations are relatively uncommon compared to the prevalence of hypertension, and are thus not the most likely etiology of hemorrhage in this patient.

B. Amyloid angiopathy [Incorrect] is a frequent cause of lobar hemorrhage, in older patients, usually over age 60. It is characterized by congophilic amyloid deposition in the media of the smaller arteries, usually at the gray-white junction.

C. Metastatic lesion [Incorrect] should also be considered in the differential diagnosis of ICH but they frequently occur at the gray-white junction and the cerebellum, rather than the basal ganglia.

D. Given the patient's history and the location of the hemorrhage, the most likely cause of the intracerebral hemorrhage (ICH) is hypertension [Correct]. Most intracerebral hemorrhages in the brain parenchyma occur in areas served by small arteries that are most prone to arteriopathy of chronic hypertension. The basal ganglia, thalamus, and brain stem are the most common locations for such bleeds. Advanced age, hypertension, cigarette smoking, and alcohol consumption are all well-known risk factors for ICH. Patients of African and Hispanic descent have a higher risk compared to Whites.

E. Cerebral aneurysm [Incorrect] may rupture, particularly in patients with hypertension, but typically cause subarachnoid hemorrhage, and not deep bleeds in the basal ganglia.

16-D

A. The constellation of symptoms is consistent with migraine with aura and not seizures. Thus, treatment with the antiepileptic agent Phenytoin [Incorrect] is not appropriate.

B. Acetaminophen [Incorrect] is not appropriate in the acute phase because the patient has not benefited from it previously.

C. Propranolol [Incorrect] is a frequently used daily medication for migraine prophylaxis. It does not work as an acute abortive agent.

D. This woman exhibits the classic symptoms of migraine with aura (classic migraine). The proposed mechanism for the visual symptoms is activation of the occipital cortex, followed by subsequent cortical spreading depression. Approximately one-third of patients experience the visual aura before the onset of the headache, which may consist of scotomas, fortification spectra, or flashing lights, which resolve after 20 to 25 minutes, followed by throbbing unilateral or bilateral headache. Patients frequently have a strong family history for the condition as in this patient. Serotonin (5HT) agonists, or the "triptans," are the mainstay for acute abortive therapy for severe migraines refractory to over-the-counter analgesics. Sumatriptan [Correct] is effective in decreasing the headache, nausea, vomiting, photophobia, and phonophobia associated with migraine.

E. Risperidone [Incorrect] is not appropriate as the visual phenomena are not part of a psychotic syndrome.

17-D

A. Head CT [Incorrect] is recommended before lumbar puncture to evaluate for possible space-occupying lesions. Other signs of space-occupying lesions include papilledema or focal neurologic deficits.

B. Lumbar puncture [Incorrect] should be performed, and opening pressure are elevated in 90% of cases. The CSF should be examined for color, cell count, protein, and glucose, as well as gram stain, bacterial, fungal, and viral cultures. Serum cultures also should be obtained.

C. EEG [Incorrect] is recommended for those who had a convulsion, or in those with persistent altered mental status, in whom subclinical seizures are suspected.

D. This young girl has classic symptoms of bacterial meningitis: fever, confusion/lethargy, headache, and neck stiffness. Eighty percent of patients have signs of meningeal irritation (e.g., nuchal rigidity and Kernig's sign). However, these signs may be absent in patients who have an altered level of consciousness, or those who are very young or very old. The presence of petechial rash points to the organism *Neisseria meningitidis,* also simply known as meningococcus. Approximately 50 to 60% of patients infected by meningococcal meningitis have the rash. The course is typically rapid, and may be associated with alteration in mental status, focal neurologic deficits, or cranial neuropathies. Although all of the diagnostic tests listed are important, they are initiated only after antibiotics are initiated. It is of paramount importance to initiate broad spectrum antibiotics [Correct] as early as possible, due to the rapid course of the disease and high mortality.

E. Blood cultures [Incorrect] should also be obtained to check for systemic and blood-borne infection.

18-C

A. MRI of the brain [Incorrect] is normal in myasthenia gravis.

B. Lumbar puncture [Incorrect] is also normal in myasthenia gravis.

C. This patient presents with symptoms that suggest myasthenia gravis, an immune-mediated attack on postsynaptic acetylcholine (ACh) receptors on the muscle via antibodies. The condition is more common in women and is characterized by fluctuating weakness and fatigability. Extraocular muscles are affected in 90% of patients, with asymmetric ocular palsies and ptosis, which become more pronounced on prolonged upgaze. Other affected areas include muscles of the larynx, pharynx, face, respiration, and limb and neck muscles. This disorder is occasionally unmasked by a concurrent infection, as in this case. The symptom severity can fluctuate throughout the day, and is usually worse at the end of the day. Weakness can be precipitated by repeated exercise.

In the emergency room, the best bedside confirmatory test is intravenous edrophonium (Tensilon) test [Correct]. Edrophonium is an acetylcholinesterase inhibitor which prolongs the action of acetylcholine. The test is positive if there is clear improvement in muscle strength of the weak muscles and typically lasts about 5 minutes. Bedside atropine should be available to anticipate for possible cholinergic side effects that may result from this test.

D. Nerve conduction studies [Incorrect] typically show decrement in muscles compound action potential on repetitive stimulation (>10% decrement) but is usually not indicated or available in the emergency room setting.

E. Muscle biopsy [Incorrect] may be performed at a later time, but is not an appropriate immediate confirmatory test.

19-B

A. Lyme disease [Incorrect] is a tick-borne infection by the spirochete *Borrelia burgdorferi,* which can cause facial nerve palsies. Patients typically give a history of hiking in the woods, tick bites, and may have a pathognomonic skin lesion, erythema migrans.

B. This man has the classic signs and symptoms of peripheral facial nerve palsy (cranial nerve VII), including weakness of the upper and lower face, loss of taste in the anterior two-thirds of the tongue, and hyperacusis (sensitivity to loud sounds). This patient also has signs of herpetic eruption of the ear, which is most likely the cause of his facial nerve palsy. This constellation of symptoms is known as Ramsay Hunt syndrome [Correct], in which the geniculate ganglion of the facial nerve is infected by varicella zoster virus (human herpes virus 3). Treatment includes acyclovir and corticosteroids.

C. Sarcoidosis [Incorrect] is a noncaseating granulomatous disease in which there is an exaggerated immune reaction mediated by T lymphocytes. Approximately 5% of patients with systemic disease may have involvement of the central nervous system, manifested by neurosarcoidosis. The facial nerve is the most commonly affected cranial nerve in neurosarcoidosis.

D. Ischemic stroke [Incorrect] typically causes an upper motor neuron pattern of facial palsy, characterized by significant weakness of the lower face, with relative sparing of the upper face, due to bilateral representation of the upper face. In a small number of patients, there is more unilateral representation of the upper face, and an upper motor neuron lesion may result in significant weakness of both the upper and lower facial muscles. Very rarely, lacunar strokes in the pons may involve the facial nerve nucleus and cause peripheral facial nerve palsy. However, these patients typically also present with contralateral hemiparesis, which is absent in this case.

E. Tumor [Incorrect], infiltration of the facial nerve such as tumors of the parotid gland, is a rare cause of facial nerve palsy. Tumors in the cerebellopontine angle or internal auditory canal may also cause facial nerve palsy, but dysfunction of other adjacent cranial nerves is also present.

20-E

A. The visual symptoms described are brief and monocular, not typical for visual auras associated with migraine [Incorrect].

B. Partial seizures [Incorrect] are not monocular. Also, occipital seizures typically present with positive symptoms, such as elemental colors or shapes, rather than loss of vision.

C. Patients with acute angle closure glaucoma [Incorrect] complain of pain in the eyes with injection, blurry vision, or halos around objects due to increased pressure. They do not usually present with transient and self-limited painless loss of vision in the descending pattern.

D. Optic neuritis [Incorrect] is frequently a manifestation of multiple sclerosis in young women, characterized by loss of visual acuity and color vision, which evolve over days. They do not resolve spontaneously over minutes.

E. This patient has amaurosis fugax [Correct] or transient monocular blindness, classically described as "curtain coming down," is caused by emboli into the retinal arteries. Occasionally, funduscopic examination may demonstrate embolic material in a branch of the central retinal artery, which is a branch of the ophthalmic artery. The ophthalmic artery is the first branch of the internal carotid artery. Emboli most frequently arise from atherosclerotic lesions at the carotid bifurcation, but may also arise from cardiac sources. Patients must undergo appropriate evaluations and treatment to minimize their subsequent risk for stroke.

credits

Austen KF, Frank MM, et al. *Samter's Immunologic Diseases*. 6th ed. Philadelphia: Lippincott Williams & Wilkins; 2001. Fig. 42.1B (42-1).

Bailey BJ, Johnson JT, et al. *Head and Neck Surgery—Otolaryngology*. 4th ed. Philadelphia: Lippincott Williams & Wilkins; 2006. Fig. 134.33 (48-1).

Becker KL, Bilezikian JP, Brenner WJ, et al. *Principles and Practice of Endocrinology and Metabolism*. 3rd ed. Philadelphia: Lippincott Williams & Wilkins; 2001. Fig. 20.9 (49-1).

Bhushan V, Le T, Pall V. *Underground Clinical Vignettes: Step 2 Neurology*. 3rd ed. Malden, MA: Blackwell Publishing; 2005. Figs. 29A (1-1), 29B (1-2), 21A (5-1), 21B (5-2), 33 (20-1), 43 (25-1), 40 (27-1), 44 (29-1), 34A (35-1), 34B (35-2), 23 (36-1), 30 (39-1), 24A (51-1), 24B (51-1), 11 (64-1), 13 (66-1), 14A (67-1), 14B (67-2), 12 (70-1), 09 (71-1).

Cohen WR. *Cherry and Merkatz's Complications of Pregnancy*. 5th ed. Philadelphia: Lippincott Williams & Wilkins Fig. 27.10 (65-2).

Eisenberg RL. *Clinical Imaging: An Atlas of Differential Diagnosis*. 4th ed. Philadelphia: Lippincott Williams & Wilkins; 2002. Figs. SK 6-2 (45-1), SK 5-1 (47-1).

Kantoff PW, et al. *Prostate Cancer: Principles & Practice*. Philadelphia: Lippincott Williams & Wilkins; 2002. Fig. 47-1 (61-1).

Keyes DC, Burstein JL, et al. *Medical Response to Terrorism: Preparedness and Clinical Practice*. Philadelphia: Lippincott Williams & Wilkins; 2004. Fig. 11.6 (41-1).

Loeser JD, Butler SH, et al. *Bonica's Management of Pain*. 3rd ed. Philadelphia: Lippincott Williams & Wilkins; 2000. Fig. 59-25 A-C (57-1).

Menkes JH, Sarnat HB, Maria BL. *Child Neurology*. 7th ed. Philadelphia: Lippincott Williams & Wilkins; 2005. Figs. 7.14 (6-1), 3.5 (13-1), I.3 (59-2).

Mills SE, et al. *Sternberg's Diagnostic Surgical Pathology*. 4th ed. Philadelphia: Lippincott Williams & Wilkins; 2004. Figs. 10-138 A-C (17-1), 10-138 G-I (21-1).

Mulholland MW, Lillemoe KD, Doherty GM, et al. *Greenfield's Surgery: Scientific Principles & Practice.* 4th ed. Philadelphia: Lippincott Williams & Wilkins; 2005. Figs. 114.13A (14-1), 114.4A (59-1), 114.2 (72-1), 114.3 (72-2).

Rowland LP. *Merritt's Neurology.* 11th ed. Philadelphia: Lippincott Williams & Wilkins; 2005. Figs. 60.4 (46-1), 46.1 (65-1), 39.4B (68-1).

Sheilds TW, et al. *General Thoracic Surgery.* 6th ed. Philadelphia: Lippincott Williams & Wilkins; 2004. Figs. 104-2A (40-1), 104-2B (40-2).

Wachter RM, Goldman L, Hollander H. *Hospital Medicine.* 2nd ed. Philadelphia: Lippincott Williams & Wilkins; 2005. Fig. 117.6 A-C (73-2).

case list

AUTOIMMUNE/ID
1. Multiple Sclerosis
2. Meningitis—Bacterial
3. Meningitis—Aseptic
4. Tuberculous Meningitis
5. Herpes Simplex Encephalitis
6. Subacute Sclerosing Panencephalitis
7. Tabes Dorsalis
8. Progressive Multifocal Leukodystrophy
9. Ramsay Hunt Syndrome

CONGENITAL
10. Cerebral Palsy
11. Wilson's Disease
12. Von Hippel–Lindau Disease
13. Friedreich's Ataxia

CRANIAL NERVE
14. Oculomotor Nerve Palsy
15. Trigeminal Neuralgia
16. Bell's Palsy

DEMENTIA
17. Alzheimer's Disease
18. Vascular Dementia
19. Wernicke-Korsakoff Syndrome
20. Normal Pressure Hydrocephalus
21. Dementia with Lewy Bodies
22. Frontotemporal Dementia (Pick's Disease)
23. Creutzfeldt–Jakob Disease

EPILEPSY
24. Status Epilepticus
25. Seizure, Grand Mal
26. Complex Partial Seizures
27. Absence Seizure
28. Febrile Seizure
29. Seizure, Metastatic Disease

HEADACHE
30. Temporal Arteritis (Giant Cell Arteritis)
31. Classic Migraine (Migraine with Aura)
32. Cluster Headache
33. Tension Headache
34. Pseudotumor Cerebri

MOVEMENT
35. Parkinson's Disease
36. Huntington's Disease
37. Gilles de la Tourette's Syndrome
38. Hemiballismus

NEUROMUSCULAR
39. Myasthenia Gravis
40. Lambert Eaton Myasthenic Syndrome—Lung Cancer
41. Botulism
42. Dermatomyositis
43. Duchenne Muscular Dystrophy
44. Myotonic Muscular Dystrophy

ONCOLOGY
45. Glioblastoma Multiforme
46. Astrocytoma
47. Meningioma
48. Acoustic Neuroma
49. Craniopharyngioma
50. Pituitary Adenoma
51. Medulloblastoma
52. Neuroblastoma

PERIPHERAL NERVE

53. Peripheral Neuropathy Due to Vincristine
54. Amyotrophic Lateral Sclerosis
55. Guillain–Barré Syndrome
56. Poliomyelitis
57. Carpal Tunnel Syndrome
58. Vitamin B_{12} Deficiency

SPINAL

59. Brown-Séquard Syndrome
60. Spinal Cord Injury
61. Spinal Cord Compression (From Metastatic Prostate Cancer)

STROKE

62. Wernicke's Aphasia
63. Broca's Aphasia
64. Stroke, Hypertensive

65. Subarachnoid Hemorrhage
66. Stroke, Left MCA Infarct
67. Stroke, Right MCA Infarct
68. Wallenberg Syndrome (Lateral Medullary Infarct or PICA Syndrome)
69. Stroke, Transient Monocular Blindness
70. Stroke, Lacunar
71. Stroke Due to Amyloid Angiopathy

TRAUMA

72. Epidural Hematoma
73. Subdural Hematoma—Acute

OTHER

74. Horner's Syndrome
75. Ménière's Disease
76. Narcolepsy

index

Absence seizures, 53–54
Acetaminophen, 66
Acetazolamide, 68
Acetylcholine function impairment, 79–80
Acetylcholinesterase inhibitor, 79–80
Achlorhydria, 115
Acoustic neuroma, 95–96
Acyclovir, 10, 18, 32, 166, 169
Adriamycin, 106
Alcoholic cerebellar degeneration, 37–38, 154, 164. *See also* Delirium tremens
Alzheimer's disease (AD), 33–34 dementia with lewy bodies v., 41–42
Amantadine, 70, 155, 164
Amaurosis fugax, 137–138, 155, 160, 165, 174
Amitriptyline, 66, 106
Amnesia. *See* Memory testing
Amyloid angiopathy, 141–142, 170
Amyloid plaques, 33–34
Amyotrophic lateral sclerosis (ALS), 107–108
Anemia, pernicious, 115–116, 163
Aneurysm, 27–28, 129–130, 171. *See also* Stroke
Anterior pituitary adenomas, 100
Antibiotics, broad spectrum, 159, 172. *See also specific antibiotic*
Anticholinergics, 2, 70, 169
Anticipation phenomenon, 88
Anticoagulation therapy, 124, 168
Antiepileptic treatment, 12, 58
Antiplatelet agents, 124, 126

Antiretroviral medications, 106
Aphasia. *See also* Speech difficulty Broca's, 125–126 Wernicke's, 123–124
Argyll-Robertson pupil, 13–14
Arteriovenous malformations, 170
Aseptic meningitis, 5–6
Aspirin, 138, 167, 168
Astrocytoma, 91–92, 163. *See also* Tumor
Ataxia, Friedreich's, 25–26
Atrial fibrillation, 156–157, 168–169
Autoimmune-mediated reaction, 109–110
Autosomal-dominant disease, 23–24, 71–72, 87–88
Autosomal-recessive disease, 25–26. *See also* X-linked recessive disorder

Babinski's sign, 25, 35–36, 107–108
Baclofen, 30
Bacterial meningitis, 3–4, 159, 172
Bell's palsy, 31–32, 166 Lyme disease feature, 156, 167, 173
Benzodiazepines, 42, 170
Benztropine, 157, 169
Beta-blockers, 62, 142, 168
Beta-interferon, 2
Blisters, ear canal (herpes zoster oticus), 17–18
Botulism, 81–82
Bradycardia, 145–146
Broca's aphasia, 125–126
Bromocriptine, 70, 100

Brown-Séquard syndrome, 117–118
Brudzinski's sign, 3–4, 7–8, 129
B_1 deficiency (Wernicke-Korsakoff syndrome), 37–38
B_{12} deficiency, 115–116, 163

Calcium-channel blocker, 168
Cancer. See also Tumor
    lung, 79–80
    medulloblastoma, 101–102, 163
    metastatic disease seizures, 57–58
    prostate, 121–122
Carbamazepine, 2, 30, 50, 52
Carbidopa, 70
Cardiac evaluation, 87–88
Cardioembolic event, 123–124, 156–157, 168
Cardiomyopathy, hypertrophic, 25–26
Carotid artery stenosis, 126, 137–138, 157, 168
Carpal tunnel syndrome, 113–114
Cataplexy, 151–152
Ceftriaxone, 4, 167, 169
Cerebral amyloid angiopathy (CAA), 141–142, 170
Cerebral palsy, 19–20
Cervical collar (soft), 153
Chemotherapy, 17–18, 80, 90, 92, 102
Cholinesterase inhibitor (physostigmine), 164
Chorea, 71–72
Cidofovir, 16
Cisplatin, 106
Clonidine, 74
Clopidogrel, 168
Coma, 38, 144
Congo red, 142
Copper excretion, 21–22
Corticosteroids, 2, 8, 10, 18, 60, 68, 78, 84, 90, 122, 166. See also Glucocorticoids; Steroids

Craniopharyngioma, 97–98
Creatine kinase, elevated, 83–84, 85–86
Creutzfeldt–Jakob disease (CJD), 45–46
Cushing reflex, 143–144
Cysts, renal polycythemia (von Hippel–Lindau disease), 23–24

Dapsone, 106
Deep tendon reflexes (DTRs)
    asymmetrically hyperactive, 1–2
    cerebral palsy, 19–20
Delirium tremens, 157, 170. See also Alcoholic cerebellar degeneration
Dementia
    Alzheimer's disease, 33–34
    Creutzfeldt–Jakob disease, 45–46
    frontotemporal, 43–44
    Huntington's disease, 71–72
    with lewy bodies, 41–42
    normal pressure hydrocephalus, 39–40
    progressive multifocal leukodystrophy, 15–16
    vascular, 35–36
Demyelination, 109–110
    multiple sclerosis, 1–2, 155, 165, 168
    progressive multifocal leukodystrophy, 15–16
Dermatomyositis, 83–84
Diabetes mellitus, 25–26, 28, 140
    insulin-dependent, 35–36
Dihydroergotamine nasal spray, 62
Diphenhydramine, 169
Dipyridamole, 168
Donepezil. See Acetylcholinesterase inhibitor
Dopamine receptor blockers, 72, 76
Down syndrome, 34
D-Penicillamine, 22
Drooling, 21–22

Dry mouth, 81–82
Duchenne muscular dystrophy, 85–86
Dystonia, 71–72

Ear canal blisters (herpes zoster oticus), 17–18
Edrophonium (Tensilon) test, 78, 159, 172
Encephalitis, 9–10, 11–12
Encephalopathy, 37–38, 45–46
Endolymphatic system, 149–150
Ependymomas, 154, 163. See also Tumor
Epidural hematoma, 143–144
Ergotamine, 64
Erythrocyte sedimentation rate (ESR), elevated, 59–60, 165
Ethambutol, 8
Ethionamide, 106
Eye/vision abnormalities, 21–22, 160, 174. See also Seizure; Stroke
    acute angle-closure glaucoma, 165
    botulism causing, 81–82
    double vision/ptosis, 77–78
    endgaze nystagmus (Wernicke-Korsakoff), 37–38
    Friedreich's ataxia, 25–26
    hemangioblastomas, 23–24
    Horner's syndrome, 147–148
    oculomotor nerve palsy, 27–28
    pseudotumor cerebri, 67–68
    ptosis, 77–78, 81–82, 147–148, 159
    tics, 73–74
    transient monocular vision loss, 137–138, 155, 160, 165, 174

Facial palsy/paralysis, 129–130, 173
    Bell's palsy, 31–32, 156, 166, 167, 173

bilateral (myasthenia gravis), 77–78, 167
    Ramsay Hunt syndrome, 17–18, 160, 173
Febrile seizure, 55–56
Fever
    chills and (herpes simplex encephalitis), 9–10
    meningitis, 3–8, 159, 172
Fluorescent treponemal antibody-absorption test (FTA-ABS), 13–14
Foot deformity, 25–26, 88
Friedreich's ataxia, 25–26
Furosemide, 68

Gabapentin, 2, 30, 66, 106
Gait unsteadiness, 85–86. See also Alcoholic cerebellar degeneration
    Friedreich's ataxia, 25–26
    medulloblastoma, 101–102, 163
    normal pressure hydrocephalus, 39–40
    spastic (cerebral palsy), 19–20
    tabes dorsalis, 13–14
    Wernicke-Korsakoff syndrome, 37–38
Galantamine. See Acetylcholinesterase inhibitor
Giant cell arteritis, 59–60, 165
Gilles de la Tourette's syndrome, 73–74
Glasgow Coma Scale (GCS), 144
Glaucoma, acute angle-closure, 165, 174
Glioblastoma multiforme (GBM), 89–90, 163
Glucocorticoids, 32. See also Corticosteroids
Gottron papules, 83–84
Gower's sign, 85–86
Grand mal seizures, 49–50
Guillain–Barré syndrome, 110

Haemophilus influenzae, 4

Haldol, 41, 169

Haloperidol, 72, 74, 76

Headache
  cluster, 63–64, 165
  intermittent right-sided (oculo-
    motor nerve palsy), 27–28
  medulloblastoma, 101–102, 163
  meningitis, 3–8, 159, 172
  migraine, 61–62, 158, 171
  new-onset (temporal arteritis),
    59–60, 165
  pseudotumor cerebri, 67–68
  severe (craniopharyngioma),
    97–98
  subarachnoid hemorrhage,
    129–130
  tension, 65–66
  von Hippel–Lindau disease,
    23–24

Hearing impairment/loss. *See also*
  Ear canal blisters (herpes
  zoster oticus)
  acoustic neuroma, 95–96
  Ramsay Hunt syndrome, 17–18,
    160, 173
  tinnitus, 149–150

Hemangioblastomas, 23–24

Hematoma, 143–146

Hemiballismus, 75–76

Hemorrhage
  intracerebral, 127–128, 158, 170
  subarachnoid, 129–130

Heparin, 140, 148, 166, 168

Herpes simplex virus (HSV)
  Bell's palsy from, 31–32, 156,
    166, 167, 173
  encephalitis, 9–10

Herpes zoster oticus, 17–18

Horner's syndrome, 64, 147–148

Huntington's disease, 71–72

Hydralazine, 106

Hydrocephalus, normal pressure,
  39–40

Hyperreflexia, progressive multifocal
  leukodystrophy, 15–16

Hypertension. *See also* Stroke
  hemiballismus, 75–76
  hypertensive stroke, 157,
    158, 170
  portal, 21–22
  vascular dementia, 35–36

Hypertensive stroke, 157, 170

Hypervolemia, 130

Immunoglobulin, 78

Insulin-dependent diabetes
  mellitus (IDDM), 35–36

Interferon, 12

Intracranial pressure (ICP),
  lumbar puncture avoidance
  with, 92

Isoniazid, 8

JC virus, 15–16

"Jerking" movements, 11–12,
  71–72

Kayser-Fleischer ring, 21–22

Kernig's sign, 3–8, 129, 159, 172

Lacrimation, 64

Lacunar stroke, 139–140

Lambert Eaton myasthenic
  Syndrome (LEMS), 79–80

Lamotrigine, 50

Lateral medullary infarction,
  135–136

Legs
  Brown-Séquard syndrome,
    117–118
  deep vein thrombosis, 163
  discomfort/fasciculations in,
    154, 163
  Guillain–Barré syndrome, 110
  hypertrophied calves, 85–86
  pain in (tabes dorsalis), 13–14
  poliomyelitis, 111–112

Lesions
  cranial nerve (Wernicke-Korsakoff syndrome), 38
  lacunar infarctions, 139–140
  metastatic, 57
  multiple periventricular white matter, 1–2, 19–20, 39–40
  neuroanatomic (lateral medullary infarction), 135–136
Levodopa, 70
Lidocaine, 64
Lithium, 64
Liver function test (LFT) abnormalities, Wilson's disease, 21–22
Lorazepam, 170
Lou Gehrig's disease, 107–108
Lumbar puncture
  meningitis, 159, 172
  Ramsay Hunt syndrome, 160, 173
Lyme disease, 156, 167, 173
Lymphocytic pleocytosis
  multiple sclerosis, 1–2, 155, 165, 168
  tabes dorsalis, 13–14
Lymphoma, 163

Magnetic resonance imaging (MRI), multiple sclerosis, 155, 165, 168
Mannitol, 10
MCA. *See* Middle cerebral artery
Medulloblastoma, 101–102, 163
Memantine, 34
Memory testing, 33–34, 36–37, 39–40, 41–42, 45–46. *See also* Dementia; Mental status altered; Speech difficulty
  retrograde v. anterograde amnesia, 36–37
Ménière's disease, 149–150, 153
Meningioma, 93–94
Meningitis, 3–8, 159, 172

Mental status altered, 157, 169–170. *See also* Memory testing; Personality changes
  bacterial meningitis, 3–4, 159, 172
  cognitive decline (dementia with lewy bodies), 41–42
  Creutzfeldt–Jakob disease, 45–46
  herpes simplex encephalitis, 9–10
  Wernicke-Korsakoff syndrome, 37–38
Methotrexate, 84
Methylprednisolone, 120
Methysergide, 64
Metoclopramide, 157, 169
Mexiletine, 88
Middle cerebral artery (MCA), 131–134
Migraine, with aura, 61–62, 158, 171
Mononuclear pleocytosis, 5–6, 9–10
Moro's reflexes, 18–19
Multiple sclerosis (MS), 1–2, 155, 165, 168
Muscle weakness, 107–108
  cataplexy, 151–152
  proximal, 84
Myasthenia gravis, 77–78, 167
Myotonic muscular dystrophy, 87–88

Naloxone, 38
Narcolepsy, 151–152
Neck
  asymmetric tonic reflexes, 18–19
  stiffness (meningitis), 3–8, 159, 172
Neuroblastoma, 103–104
Neurofibrillary tangles (Alzheimer's disease), 33–34
Neurosyphilis, 14, 163
Nimodipine, 130

Nonsteroidal anti-inflammatory drugs (NSAIDs), 62, 66. *See also* Steroids
Normal pressure hydrocephalus, 39–40
Nuchal rigidity, meningitis, 3–8, 159, 172

Obsessive-compulsive disorder, 73–74
Oculomotor nerve palsy, 27–28
Olfactory hallucinations, 9–10
Oligoclonal bands, 1–2, 11–12
Oligodendrocytes, progressive multifocal leukodystrophy, 15–16
Optic neuritis, 174
Oxygen, 38, 64

Palsy
   Bell's, 156, 166, 167
   Ramsay Hunt syndrome, 160, 173
Pancoast's lung tumor, 148
Pancreas, von Hippel–Lindau disease, 23–24
Papovavirus, 15–16
Parkinson's disease, 69–70
   dementia with lewy bodies v., 41–42
   Risperidone contraindicated for, 164
Penicillin, 14, 22
Personality changes, 21–22, 35–36, 43. *See also* Mental status altered
Petit mal seizures, 53–54
Phenytoin, 10, 30, 50, 52, 106, 169, 170
Physostigmine. *See* Cholinesterase inhibitor
PICA syndrome, 135–136
Pick's disease, 43–44
Pituitary adenoma, 99–100

Pituitary hypofunction, craniopharyngioma symptom, 97–98
Plaques
   amyloid (Alzheimer's disease), 33–34
   CNS white matter, 1–2, 19–20, 39–40
Plasmapheresis, 110
Pleocytosis
   lymphocytic, 1–2, 13–14, 155, 165, 168
   mononuclear, 5–6, 9–10
Poliomyelitis, 111–112
Polycythemia, von Hippel–Lindau disease, 23–24
Polymerase chain reaction (PCR), positive, 9–10, 15–16
Prednisone, 64, 68, 166. *See also* Corticosteroids
Premature birth, cerebral palsy associated with, 19–20
Prion, 45–46
Prochloperazine, 157
Progressive multifocal leukodystrophy (PML), 15–16
Propranolol, 170
Prostate cancer, metastatic, 121–122
Protein level, elevated
   Guillain–Barré syndrome, 109–110
   herpes simplex encephalitis, 9–10
   Ramsay Hunt syndrome, 17–18, 160, 173
   tabes dorsalis, 13–14
Pseudotumor cerebri, 67–68
Ptosis, 77–78, 81–82, 147–148, 159
Pyrazinamide, 8
Pyridostigmine, 78, 80

Radiation therapy, 100, 122
Radiosurgery, stereotactic, 96
Radiotherapy, 90, 92, 102

Ramsay Hunt syndrome, 17–18, 160, 173
Rapid plasma reagin (RPR), positive (tabes dorsalis), 13–14
Rash, erythematous, 83–84
Reflexes
  asymmetric tonic, 18–19
  deep tendon, 1–2, 19–20
  hyperreflexia (progressive multifocal leukodystrophy), 15–16
  primitive (vascular dementia diagnostic), 35–36
Renal disorders, von Hippel–Lindau disease, 23–24
Retrograde amnesia, 36–37
Rifampin, 8
Riluzole, 108
Risperidone, 164
Rivastigmine. *See* Acetylcholinesterase inhibitor
Romberg sign, tabes dorsalis, 13–14

Sarcoidosis, 173
Schilling test, 115, 116
Schwannoma, 95–96
Seizure, 174. *See also* Eye/vision abnormalities
  absence, 53–54
  astrocytoma complication, 92
  complex partial, 51–52
  febrile, 55–56
  glioblastoma multiforme, 89–90
  grand mal, 49–50
  herpes simplex encephalitis, 9–10
  metastatic disease, 57–58
  status epilepticus, 47–48
Selegiline, 70
Sensory nerve impairment (herpes simplex encephalitis), 9–10
Shingles, 17–18
Skull fracture, 143–144
Sleepiness. *See also* Seizure
  on awakening/confusion, 153, 162

excessive (narcolepsy), 151–152
REM disorder (dementia with lewy bodies), 41–42
Speech difficulty, 43–44. *See also* Memory testing
  Broca's aphasia, 125–126
  "gibberish" (Wernicke's aphasia), 123–124
  paraphasic errors (herpes simplex encephalitis), 9–10
  slow and dysarthric (progressive multifocal leukodystrophy), 15–16
  slurring (Wilson's disease), 21–22
Spinal cord
  Brown-Séquard syndrome, 117–118
  compression of, 121–122
  degeneration of (B12 deficiency), 115–116, 163
  injury, 120–121
Status epilepticus, 47–48
Stereotactic radiosurgery, 96
Steroids, 4, 58. *See also* Corticosteroids; Nonsteroidal anti-inflammatory drugs; *specific type*
Streptococcus pneumoniae, 3–4
Stroke, 156–157, 168, 173. *See also* Aneurysm; Transient monocular blindness
  amyloid angiopathy causing, 141–142, 170
  hypertensive, 127–128, 157, 158, 170
  intracerebral hemorrhage from, 127–128, 158, 170
  lacunar, 139–140
  left MCA infarction, 131–132
  right MCA infarction, 133–134
Subacute sclerosing panencephalitis (SSPE), 11–12
Subarachnoid hemorrhage, 129–130

Subdural hematoma, acute,
    145–146
Sumatriptan, 62, 64
Sustained clonus (progressive
    multifocal leukodystrophy),
    15–16
Syphilis, neuro-, 14, 163

Tabes dorsalis, 13–14
Tachycardia
    bacterial meningitis, 3–4,
        159, 172
    herpes simplex encephalitis, 9–10
Tachypnea, 9–10
Taxol, 106
Temporal arteritis, 59–60, 165
Thalamotomy, 76
Thiamine deficiency (Wernicke-
    Korsakoff syndome),
    37–38, 163
Thymectomy, 78
Topiramate, 50
Transient monocular blindness,
    137–138, 155, 160, 165, 174
Treponema pallidum, 14, 163
Trientine, 22
Trigeminal neuralgia, 29–30
Tuberculous meningitis, 7–8
Tumor, 173. See also Cancer
    acoustic neuroma, 95–96
    astrocytoma, 91–92
    craniopharyngioma, 97–98
    ependymomas, 154, 163
    glioblastoma multiforme,
        89–90, 163
    lymphoma, 163
    medulloblastoma, 101–102, 163
    meningioma, 93–94
    neuroblastoma, 103–104
    Pancoast's lung, 148
    pituitary adenoma, 99–100
    spinal cord, 117–118

Tzanck smear, positive (Ramsay
    Hunt syndrome), 17–18,
    160, 173

Urinary incontinence, 13–14,
    39–40. See also Copper
    excretion

Valproic acid, 50, 62
Vancomycin, 4
Vascular dementia, 35–36
Venereal Disease Research
    Laboratory (VDRL), 13
Verapamil, 62, 64
Vertigo, Ménière's disease,
    149–150, 153
Vincristine, peripheral neuropathy
    from, 105–106
Vision. See Eye/vision
    abnormalities
Vitamin B12 deficiency, 163
Voltage gated calcium channels
    (VGCC), 80
von Hippel–Lindau disease,
    23–24

Wallenberg syndrome, 135–136,
    148
Warfarin, 124, 148, 166
Wernicke-Korsakoff syndrome,
    37–38. See also Wernicke's
    aphasia
Wernicke's aphasia, 123–124
Wilson's disease, 21–22

X-linked recessive disorder,
    85–86. See also Autosomal-
    recessive disease

Zinc, Wilson's disease
    management, 22
Zonisamide, 50